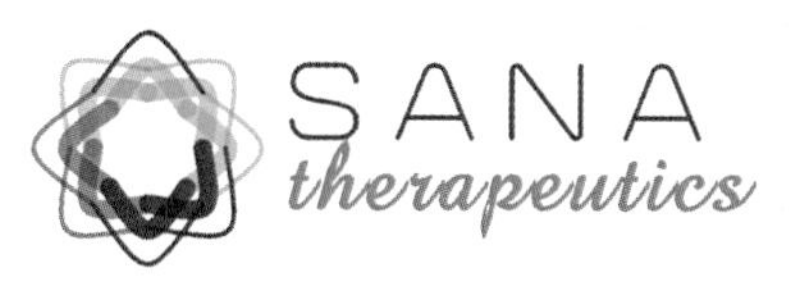

The Avazzia Life Genesis

Official User's Guide

Getting Started
& Protocol Guidebook

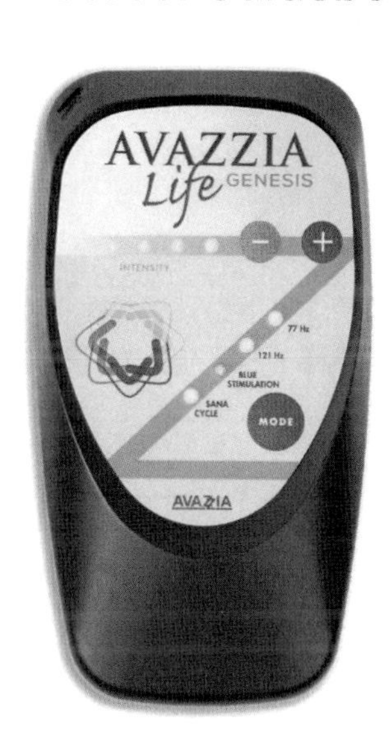

Dr. John Haché, DNM, PhD | Dr. Lorry Haché, PsyD | Rob Vanbergen, HHP

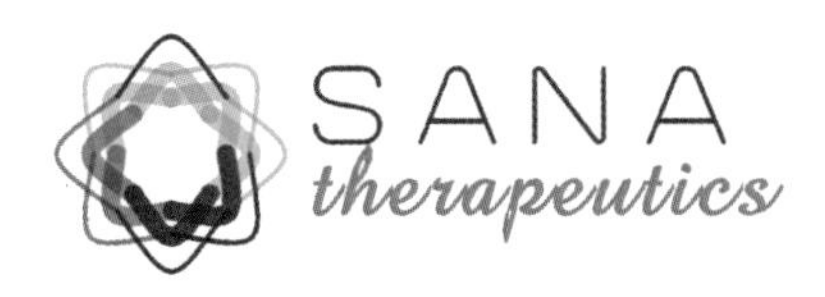

AUTHORS
Dr. John Haché, DNM, PhD
Dr. Lorry Haché, PsyD
Rob Vanbergen, HHP

DISCLAIMER

Statements within this book have not been evaluated by the Food and Drug Administration. This product is not intended to diagnose, treat, cure, or prevent any disease. The products described here are not intended to diagnose, treat, cure or prevent any disease. You should always ask your doctor before using any products.

CONTENTS

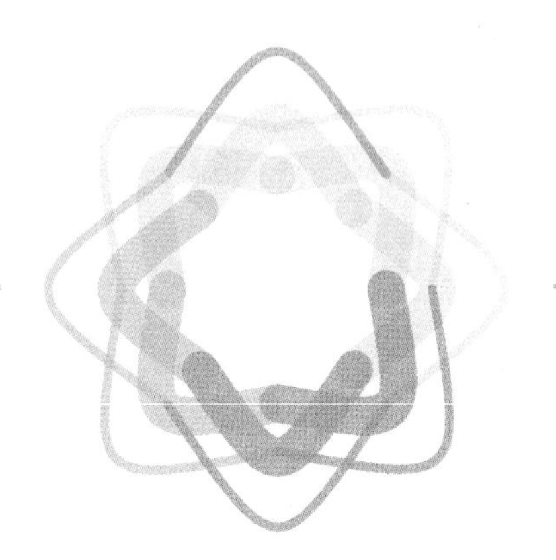

INTRODUCTION

If you are reading this, then you've taken the first step onto the path of what will undoubtedly be a phenomenal health journey.

Congratulations!

Here at Pain Free For Life, we've been involved in Microcurrent Therapy for decades. It's our "thing" and so we feel confident that we know what our clients need to get results. This is why we created the Avazzia Life Genesis. The Genesis is packed with the latest features and has been developed with your healing in mind. Ease of use was at the forefront of its development and because of this the Genesis has been designed to treat you automatically, without any knowledge of frequencies, your body's specific needs, or any extensive training. This device's biofeedback capabilities will also help to make sure that your body can work with your brain, and the device, to create an unstoppable trio that can trigger the appropriate healing process and move you towards pain resolution.

This book will serve as a start-up guide, while also teaching you some advanced techniques. You will likely be referring back to the book for quite some time until you learn how things work, however, it is just the beginning. With your device purchase you will receive 60 days access to our Hache Protocol Private Membership, which includes advanced training videos for a variety of conditions, and access to community and one-on-one support.

> If you haven't signed up yet, and you don't have the sign-up card in your device package, then please contact our support team toll-free at 1-888-758-0851, we'll be happy to send you an access link.

Also keep in mind that our entire team is here to help you. We don't expect you to go through this journey alone. Let us know however we may be of assistance.

Here's to a Pain Free Life!

The Contents of Your Kit

If you purchased the Classic Kit you will have access to the device itself, as well as a small pouch to carry it in, and some conductive pads. With the combination of its built-in electrodes and these sticky pads the Genesis can perform most techniques without any additional accessories – however the additional accessories found in the Deluxe Kit have a lot of value. In this section we will cover what should be found in your kit, and the general applications of each attachment.

Please keep in mind that all of our accessories cross between devices, so if you ever opt to upgrade your Genesis to an Evolution, or a more advanced device, your accessories will all still be compatible.

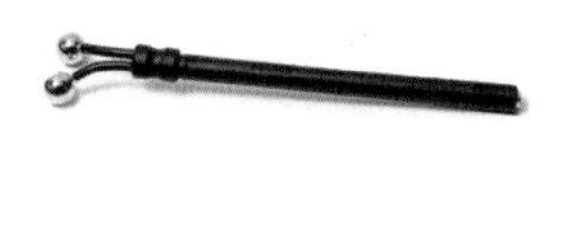

Y ELECTRODE (DELUXE KIT ONLY)

The most popular Avazzia accessory across all devices. This accessory allows for extended reach, while also enabling better contouring of the electrode, and smoother painting action. You will find for most of your general treatments, the Y Electrode will be the primary tool of choice.

PENCIL ELECTRODE (DELUXE KIT ONLY)

The improved Sana Pencil Electrode is in this kit to allow you to stimulate meridians through acupuncture points to rebalance the body's energy and help provide relief from a variety of conditions.

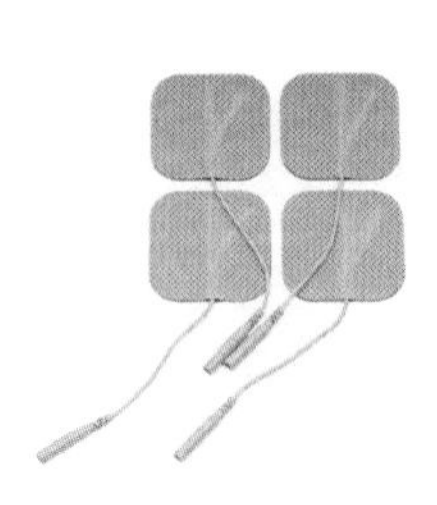

2"X 2" CONDUCTIVE PADS (BOTH KITS)

The standard conductive pads. These pads are used to treat areas through what we call "Passive Treatment". By placing the pads on an area, one out and one in, then you can treat an area while performing other tasks or resting.

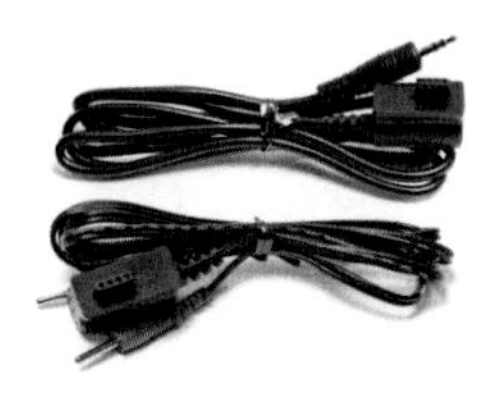

WIRES

You'll find you have a standard plug lead wire (Deluxe Kit) for your Y Electrode and Pencil Electrode, and a red/black lead wire (Both Kits) for your conductive pads.

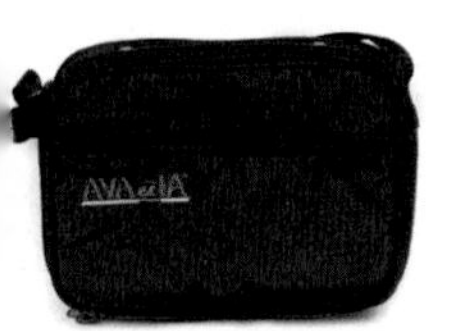

CARRY CASE (DELUXE KIT)

Your kit will have come in a medium carry case capable of containing all of the attachments and the device in a safe and secure way.

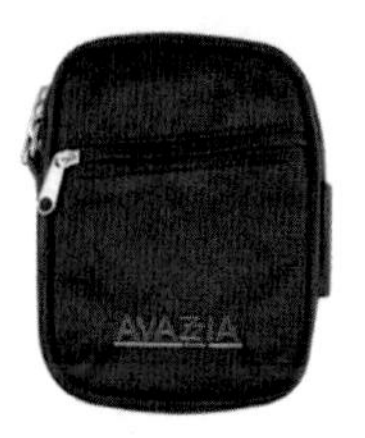

ZIPPER POUCH (CLASSIC KIT)

Your Classic Kit will include a small zipper pouch with a belt loop for safe storage of your device, wires, and conductive pads. If you decide to get a Y Electrode at any point there is a small loop on the Zipper Pouch to slot the Y Electrode into.

Getting Started – Quick Start Guide

The first thing you will need to do is to put batteries in the device. Slide open the battery cover on the back, and insert 2x AA Batteries as indicated. It is important to not use rechargeable batteries in Avazzia machines.

Refer to the diagram below for navigation. Everything is as indicated. First you slide the power button on the left side into the ON position. You will hear an audible beep, and an LED light will come on, fixed on the first frequency: 77 Hz

You can press the mode button to switch your device between modes. One press will move it down the line, and when it hits the last one (Sana Cycle) one press of the mode button will bring it back to the top.

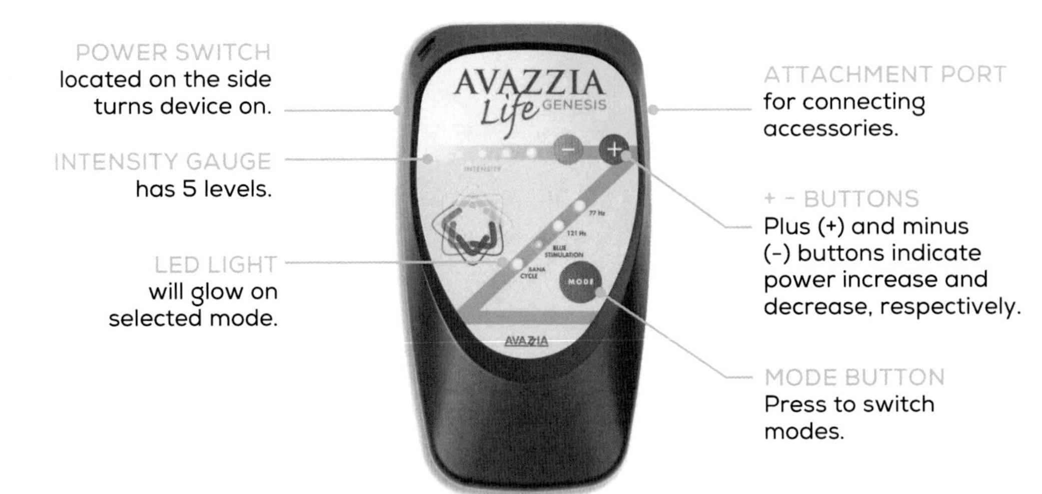

When you are on the mode you want, place the built-in rear electrodes on the skin, and hold down the power button to increase the power to the point where you can feel a tingling sensation, but which is not painful or uncomfortable. We will refer to this as a "Comfortable Power Level" throughout much of the literature. This power level is indicated in the top left of the unit by an Intensity Gauge - but the power level is always relative to you being able to comfortably feel it.

Please be aware that as the device works, it is normal to need to decrease the power as treatment progresses, and this should be seen as a sign of success. More intensity is NOT better, less is just as effective.

TO TREAT PAIN AND INFLAMMATION RIGHT OUT OF THE BOX

- Press the mode button to switch to Blue Stimulation*
- Place the electrode (Built-in Electrodes or Y Electrode) a few inches away from the area of pain, and hold down the power increase button until the device is at a Comfortable Power Level.

- Next you will need to drag the electrode across the area of pain applying gentle pressure. You are looking for the movement to be smooth. If it gets stuck or you feel what may be described as "Sticky Areas", or you see areas of prominent redness on the skin, then you have found what we refer to as an Active Zone.
- You want to continue to move the device across the active zone in all directions in order to work out the inflammatory pockets.
- This should take no longer than 15 minutes to notice a substantial difference.

*If the area is too small to drag the electrode around, then you should instead set it to 121 Hz, and hold it in place on the area of complaint.

Device Modes

The Avazzia Life Genesis is a phenomenally flexible home use microcurrent machine, with the unparalleled ability to automatically treat the user. It has four modes, each chosen for their unique capabilities. This section of the book will serve to do just that be providing you with a chart of the frequencies contained within the programs, and the general uses that they will have when treating based off of studies into the effects of these particular frequencies.

MODE NAME	FREQUENCY RANGE	PULSES	MODULATION	DOSING CAPABILITY
77 Hz	77 Hz	1	Off	Yes
General Uses: Scar Tissue, Soft Tissue Repair, Dosing/Zeroing				
121 Hz	121 Hz	1	On (3:1)	No
General Uses: Small areas of inflammation and pain, Little Wings, New Injuries				
Blue Stimulation	22-163 Hz	1-5	Off	No
General Uses: Generation of ATP, Electro-Acupuncture, Auriculotherapy, Meridian Work, Organ Deficiency, Treating Large Areas of Inflammation and pain				
Sana Cycle	Variable	Variable	Variable	No
General Uses: The perfect self-treatment. Sana Cycle is a unique proprietary combination of each frequency set designed to automatically treat an area over a 6 minute cycle.				

Using Accessories

If you have purchased the recommended Deluxe Kit, then you will have many attachments to choose from. Using these attachments is simple. On the right side of the device is a rectangular portal. This portal accepts the rectangular end of the wires included in your kit. This rectangular end is called a "4-Pin" by Avazzia.

With your device turned off, insert the wire's single or red/black pins to the accessory of choice and plug the wire's rectangular end into the Genesis.

That's it! Now rather than emit current from the built-in electrodes, the device will transfer all output into the accessories.

It is worth noting that the accessories using the Red/Black leadwire will require both pieces to make contact with the body, in order for the circuit to be complete.

Using a PEMF

One of the massive benefits to our Avazzia technology is that with the addition of an attachment you can transform your output from Microcurrent to Pulsed Electro Magnetic Fields (PEMFs), and whatever else comes in the future.

THE PEMF ACCESSORIES ARE:

- THE VIAQI: The ViaQi is a handheld, targeted PEMF device which focuses the energy through a special crystal to force the amplified energy into the body penetrating 12"- 24" or more.

  The advantages of PEMFs include lack of active sensation (due to the passive energy field), and penetration through clothing, casts, braces, etc.

  The ViaQi's ability to target very precise areas or treat from a distance makes it an extremely valuable addition to your collection.

  The ViaQi is powered by both a Tesla Coil and a Merkaba Crystal and can be detected by EMF meters when powered on (Always use MAX power when operating a ViaQi).

- QIWAVE (2 SIZES): These are mats that you can sit on, sleep on, lean against, or place between 2 people to treat both at the same time. The small has 2 tesla coils and the large has 3. Without the crystal focus they are weaker than the ViaQi, but easier to use and hands-free for convenience, covering a larger surface area. They penetrate up to 12" but are rarely detectable by an EMF sensor.

When using these attachments, they have their own special wires, but connect in just the same way as standard attachments. The one difference in using them, is that we ALWAYS max out our power levels when operating the devices.

The reason is that there is no discomfort, and it ensures maximum output across the devices.

Access your Online Training (Advanced Techniques)

Beyond the protocols in this book, there are a variety of advanced techniques. With your device (Standalone or Kit) you should have received information on a card regarding how to access your Two Free Months in our Private Membership Portal. Here you will receive access to tons of video content dedicated to helping you get started with your Genesis, as well as learning some of these advanced techniques.

Our Private Member's Community allows us to answer any questions in real time, and you get not only our input, but input from all sorts of therapists, and veteran Microcurrent users. We highly recommend you take advantage of your two free months in the membership – there is so much you can get out of it.

If this was missing from your equipment, please contact us at Support@PainFreeForLife.com and we will help you out.

Explaining Active Zones

In the getting started guide, we briefly mentioned Active Zones. These areas are primary pathway blockage sites and are often the source of pain, discomfort, and health concerns. Using the Genesis you will be able to work through these active zones, break them apart, and restore communication and harmony to the body. This can be done with any frequency, but frequencies over 100 Hz work best. This would be Blue Stimulation in the Genesis. 121 Hz only overshadows Blue Stimulation in cases of extremely small active zones where painting is not possible.

INDICATIONS OF AN ACTIVE ZONE INCLUDE:

- COLOR (Redness OR White spots among the red)
- SOUND (Your device's sound will change, or sometimes cut out completely)
- STICKINESS (The device will get stuck, or offer significant resistance to the treatment)
- SENSITIVITY OF THE SKIN (The skin in an area will either not feel the current, or be extremely sensitive to it)

Regardless of how you tackle it, the goal is to eliminate the active zone to restore normal function to the area.

Many of the protocols on the following pages will refer to "active zones" and clearing them, now you know what they are.

Dosing & Zeroing

Dosing and Zeroing are terms that up until now, you may not have ever heard before. Many treatments with the Genesis can be completed without ever needing to Dose or Zero, but learning how can help with a variety of advanced techniques, as well as any stubborn problems.

The technology is fully capable of establishing a biofeedback connection – talking with the brain in order to involve it in the healing process. In this way we can draw the attention of our body to a problem that it may have previously forgotten about. On the professional model devices, we have a screen, and that screen can help us get further involved by bringing in a concept called initial reactions in which we can directly measure the electrical conductivity and resistance of areas of the skin to determine issues prior to initiating communication. Contrary to popular belief, we can figure this out with the Genesis as well, only it is done in a bit more of a convoluted way.

In this section of the book we will teach you how to take initial reactions (IR), how to Dose, and how to Zero, with your Genesis device, as well as how to complete a DZS cycle. Moreover, we'll give examples of situations in which performing a DZS cycle will be more beneficial than just jumping straight to treatment.

WHAT DOES DOSING AND ZEROING MEAN?

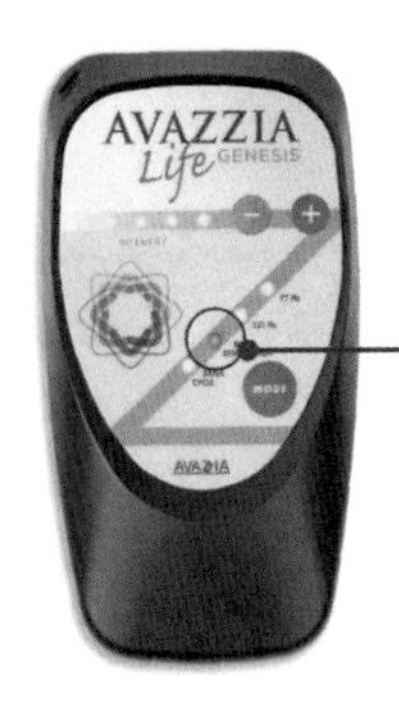

Dosing Definition: Dosing is us establishing a communication line to the brain. If your brain is a house, successfully "dosing" is knocking on the front door.
Look for the blue light to complete dosing.

Zero Definition: Zeroing is our brain accepting the communication attempt. If Dosing is us knocking on the door, Zeroing is our brain answering the door. If we successfully "dose" an area first, and then follow up with a "zero", then we have brought the brain into the healing equation.

Look for the blue light and all orange lights to complete zeroing.

If all orange lights flash before the blue light appears the attempt was NOT successful and must be repeated.

The Genesis contains Dosing and Zeroing functionality in its 77 Hz mode. This only applies when fixed in 77 Hz, and not when exposed to 77 Hz in Sana Cycle.

Dosing

To prepare the device to Dose set it to 77 Hz and to a comfortable power level, place the device on the area you wish to Dose, and hold it in place. You are waiting for the Blue LED on Blue Stimulation to light up and hold Blue. When it does you have successfully dosed the area.

If you are trying to determine the "worst" of multiple problem areas, count the seconds from placement on the skin to successful Dose (blue light appears). This is your Dose Reading and can be compared to others in a series for more advanced protocols.

Zero

Taking the device to a Zero or 'Z' is simply an extension of dosing. To accomplish this we need to continue holding the device in the same spot after it Doses, at which point we are able to allow it to continue towards 'Z'. When the Blue LED light is lit up from the dose, you will be waiting for the other three mode buttons to light up yellow. This will signal a successful Zero cycle. Please keep in mind that achieving a Zero after a dose can take several minutes.

If comparing multiple areas, you will only be Zeroing the highest Dose reading and completing all doses in a series. If doing more than 1 series, count the seconds until the Zero completes for your Zero Reading.

Stimulate

Once we have completed our Dose and our Zero in sequence, we want to stimulate the point. Press the mode button to switch the device to Blue Stimulate, adjust the power to comfortable, and treat for two minutes by holding the electrode in place.

Following the three above steps signals the completion of a Dose/Zero/Stimulate (DZS) cycle.

Note: For advanced protocols, only stimulate the highest Zero reading among multiple series.

WHEN WOULD YOU WANT TO DZS?

Not all the time, but on occasion. It's easy to fall into the trap of thinking that DZS is the best thing since sliced bread, and needs to be done all the time to get anything done. That simply isn't true. Think of DZS as a method of dealing with a stubborn problem when nothing else is working. Taking an area through the DZS cycle will establish a connection with the brain, and collaborate with it to get its attention and address the problem.

Apart from certain protocols that require it, DZS is useful to break through a metaphorical hard shell that has formed over a chronic pain area as well as brand new injuries.

Its real function is to command the attention of the body and brain. Think of standard treatments as a method of calmly asking for the body's attention, and DZS as you snapping your fingers in front of its face!

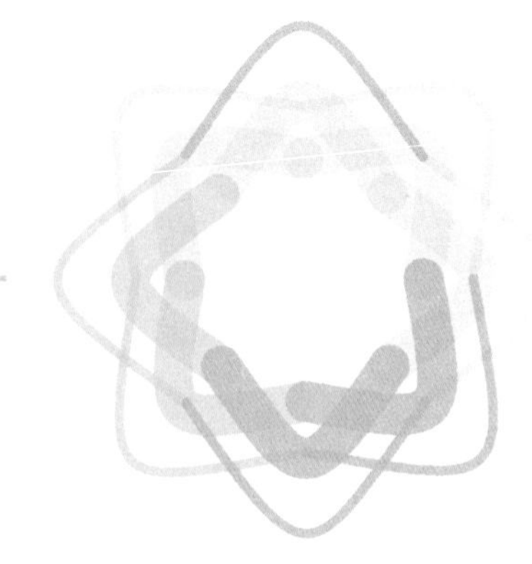

PROTOCOLS

There are many treatment protocols depending on the condition at hand, and many conditions may benefit from some over others. Remember that however you look at it, your treatment may require slightly different approaches. Every patient is different. This book contains a series of Standard Protocols, our standard protocols focus on pain resolution, and working with the body to resolve mechanical issues – before we get to the standard protocols, the Sana Cycle treatment is explained and can substitute many of the following treatments. All protocols here can be completed with the Avazzia Life Genesis device.

If a particular protocol is NOT working for you,
please contact us at Support@PainFreeForLife.com

More often than not human error is the reason that results are not being achieved, and if the issue it not human error, we can adjust the protocol accordingly to ensure that you get the results you need.

SANA CYCLE PROTOCOL – AUTOMATIC TREATMENT

The Sana Cycle Protocol was designed for ease of use and encompasses the basic rules of microcurrent therapy which are: 1) Clear Scars to open blocked pathways; 2) Reduce Inflammation to remove pain and prevent further damage; 3) Regenerate tissue by helping the body to heal itself and rebuild long-term damage.

Sana Cycle does it all with limited intervention from the user.

Wherever the area of complaint may be, place one conductive pad on the problem area, and another a few inches away. Many people opt to use conductive garments or other attachments instead. The goal is to box in the area for treatment.

Follow these steps:

1. Stick conductive pads on the area of discomfort according to the Pain Trigger Points charts in the back of this book.

2. Set your device to Sana Cycle

3. Adjust the power to a comfortable power level

4. Allow the device to treat for 6 minutes. A series of audible tones will ring and all the mode LED lights will flash when treatment is complete.

5. Treatment is complete!

Sana Cycle can be repeated as needed.

If one Cycle makes a difference great, you can stop. If not, we often recommend 2-3 complete Sana Cycles over treatment session. Check for improvement after each cycle.

Usually 1-2 treatments per day are plenty. More is not necessarily better: the body needs time to process the information between sessions.

Avoid doing more than 5 treatment sessions in one day per area.

STANDARD PROTOCOLS

Basic Pain Relief Techniques

What follows is a short series of basic pain relief protocols that involve combinations of the basic techniques we have discussed in this book to tackle general pain in specific areas. These are not meant to restrict you, but rather to act us guidelines to employ the basics of microcurrent therapy on typical areas of pain.

While treating, remember the general painting rules for active zones.

LOWER BACK PAIN

One of the most common complaints when it comes to pain is Lower Back Pain. Our body is constantly under stress, and it is estimated that up to 80% of people will deal with Chronic Back Pain at some time in their life.

The Genesis is equipped to deal with Lower Back Pain. Follow the protocol method below.

Treatment Method: Painting*

Set your device to Blue Stimulation

1. Adjust the power to a comfortable level
2. Paint (move the electrode back and forth) horizontally on either side of the spine as pictured.
3. Work out any active zones you find

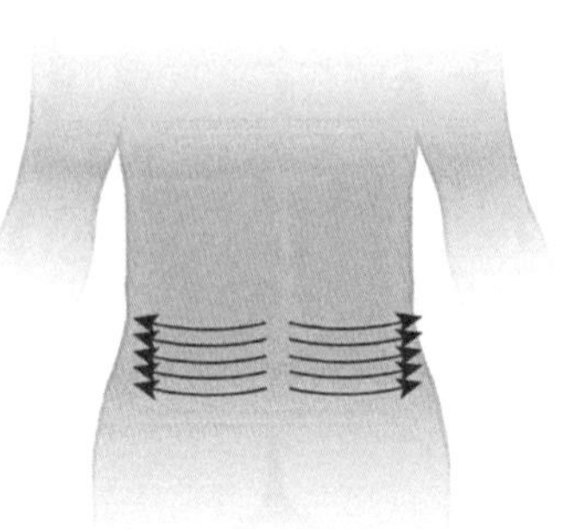

*Note: If you want to treat passively (or treat yourself), try placing a pair of conductive pads, one on either side of the spine, or using a Conductive Adjustable Back Belt and running 121 Hz

NECK PAIN

Another common type of pain experienced by people is neck pain. One effective method to treating the neck is to use the Little Wings technique detailed on page 22. For pain that is not relieved through performing Little Wings, you want to follow this simple treatment

Method 1: Stationary Treatment*

1. Set the device to 121 Hz
2. Adjust the power to a comfortable level
3. Place the Electrode on the highest point of pain
4. Hold it in place for 3 minutes
5. Treat the exact same spot on the opposite side of the neck
6. Switch to Blue Stimulation, and treat for another 5 minutes.

> *If you would prefer, you can place a conductive pad on the highest point of pain and then one on the opposite side of the neck. Run 121 Hz as above, and follow it up with Blue Stimulation. Many people prefer the Neck Wrap for frequent neck treatments.

Method 2: Painting

1. Set the device to 350 Hz
2. Adjust the power to a comfortable level
3. Begin to paint the area, paying particular attention to active zones, moving in a direction as indicated on the diagram to the left in the following order: 1 Yellow, 2 Orange, 3 Red, 4 Blue. Note how you are effectively working around that point of pain in the center of the grid.

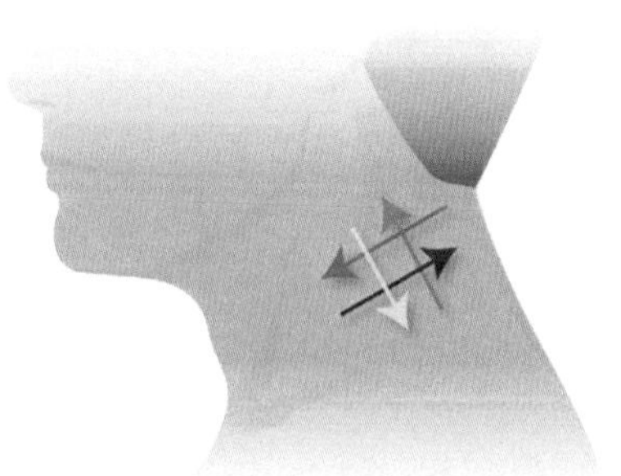

4. Be sure to work out active zones.
5. Switch to Blue Stimulation and treat for 3 minutes in the same way.
6. Look for improved flexibility and reduced pain. If the pain has moved repeat the treatment on the new area of pain.

JAW PAIN

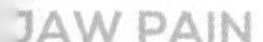

Jaw pain is another common type of pain which can be debilitating. Using these simple microcurrent treatments can help provide massive relief, or even resolve the problem.

The primary treatment for Jaw Pain is to perform the Six Points protocol detailed below. After this you should treat it with the following method.

Treatment Method: Painting

1. Set your device to Blue Stimulation
2. Adjust the power to a comfortable level
3. Place the electrode on the point of pain
4. Paint backwards – slowly- from the point of pain to the ear, working out any active zones.
5. Paint the entire jawline and cheek area slowly to provide relief.
6. Repeat on the opposite side.

SIX POINTS

The six points technique treats the six exit points of the Trigeminal Nerve for optimum pain relief of the face and jaw. It is also effective for improving conditions such as Bells Palsy and Trigeminal Neuralgia. This treatment can be repeated up to three times per day.

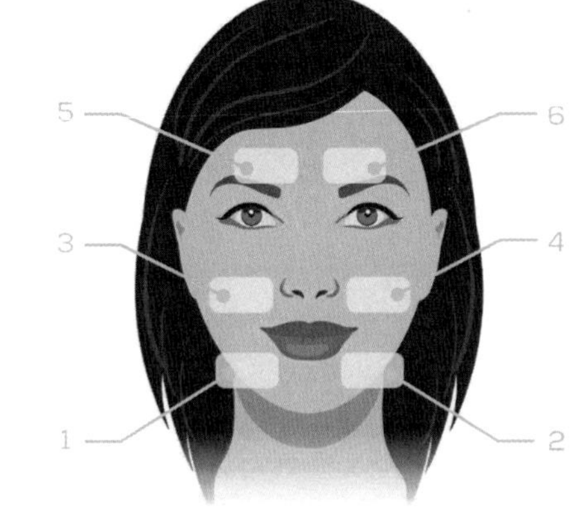

1. Set mode to 77 Hz
2. Set to comfortable power level
3. Dose each point on the chart from 1 to 6, counting or recording the seconds until the Blue LED light appears.
4. When all 6 Doses are complete return to the point with the highest Dose number and wait for a Zero.
5. Change mode to Blue Stimulate and treat for 2 minutes on the spot you Zeroed.

Recommended Attachments: This can be done with or without accessories, the Y Electrode that is included in the Deluxe Kit or Face Electrode due to its small form, and reach, will make this technique easier on your arm, but also make it easier to conform to specific points.

SHOULDER PAIN

Upper back pain is usually the result of posture, or a lack of alignment, but sometimes we just have pain there. To treat Upper Back discomfort with the Genesis we focus primarily on the point of pain with the following methods. To effectively treat pain we need a mode that operates above 100hz, proceed as follows:

Method 1:

1. Set the device to Blue Stimulation mode, place the electrode on the skin, and adjust the power to a comfortable level

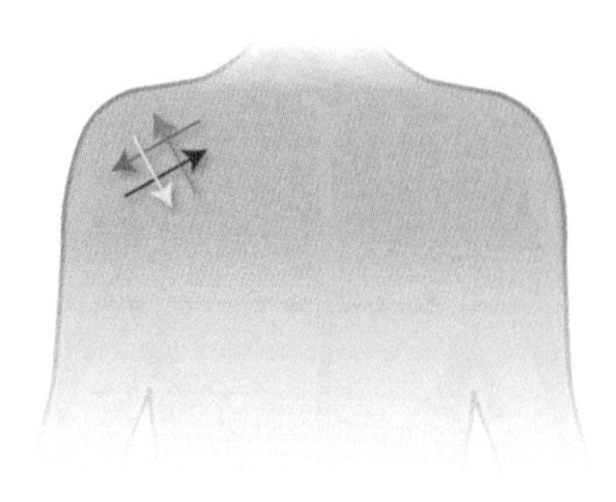

2. Begin to paint the area, paying particular attention to active zones, moving in a direction as indicated on the diagram to the left in the following order: 1 Yellow, 2 Orange, 3 Red, 4 Blue. Note how you are effectively working around that point of pain in the center of the grid.

3. Repeat step 2 in the same area on the opposite side. Check for improvement every 2-3 minutes. Treat until you notice a reduction in pain, or until 15-20 minutes has passed. Be sure to stay hydrated.

Method 2:

1. Using either the conductive pads (a pad on either side of the point of pain), or the built-in electrodes directly on the point of pain, set your device to 121 hz and adjust the power to a comfortable level.

2. If your pain is recent, switch your device to 121 hz mode, and hold it on the area, or allow the conductive pads to do their work. Leave this for 15-20 minutes. check for improvement every 2-3 minutes.

3. If your pain is chronic, and has existed for a while, then use conductive pads and run a Sana Cycle on the area. Leave this for 15-20 minutes. Check for improvement between each Cycle.

4. Move your shoulder around to see if the pain has returned, or moved.

5. If it has returned, switch to Blue Stimulation and hold it on the area for 2 minutes.

6. If the pain has moved, move to method 1 above and treat for 10 minutes.

*If these basic methods fail, we recommend attempting the "Little Wings" protocol to provide relief for shoulder pain.

WRIST

Wrist pain is often caused by sprains or fractures from sudden injuries. But wrist pain can also result from long-term problems, such as repetitive stress, arthritis and carpal tunnel syndrome.

Method 1:

1. Set the device to Blue Stimulation mode and adjust the power to a comfortable level.

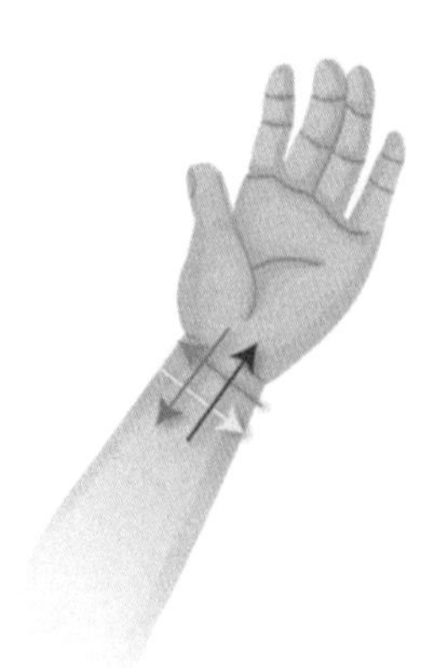

2. Begin to paint the area, paying particular attention to active zones, moving in a direction as indicated on the diagram to the right in the following order: 1 Yellow, 2 Orange, 3 Red, 4 Blue. Note how you are effectively working around that point of pain in the center of the grid.

3. Treat until you notice a reduction in pain, or until 15-20 minutes has passed. Be sure to stay hydrated. Repeat step 2 in the same area on the opposite side. Check for improvement every 2-3 minutes.

Method 2:

1. Using the conductive pads, place one on the palm, and one on the point of pain on the wrist.

2. If your pain is recent, switch your device to 121 hz mode, and hold it on the area, or allow the conductive pads to do their work. Leave this for 15-20 minutes.

3. If your pain is chronic, and has existed for a while, then run a Sana Cycle on the area.

4. Move your wrist around in a circular motion to see if the pain has returned, or moved.

5. If it has returned or there is no improvement, repeat step 3 with pads on the elbow instead.

6. If the pain has moved, move to method 1 above and treat for 10 minutes.

KNEE

Knee pain covers pain, swelling, or sensitivity in one or both knees. The cause of your knee pain can determine the symptoms you experience. Many conditions can cause or contribute to chronic knee pain, and many treatments exist. Each person's experience with knee pain will be very different, and there is a variety of different approaches to dealing with it using the Genesis.

Method 1: The simplest, and often most effective, way to treat knee pain is to place the Y Electrode behind the knee and bend the leg to hold it in place. Run 121 Hz at a comfortable power level for 3-5 minutes. This is effective because most nerve clusters and blood flow originate here and pain felt in the front of the knee is most often referred from the back. We want to address the source, not the symptom.

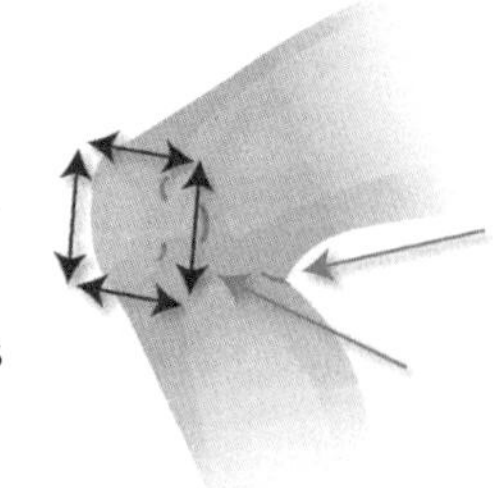

Note: Consider treating the opposite knee also to address any compensation inflammation.

Method 2: Set your device to Blue Stimulation at a comfortable power level. Paint around the patella (knee cap) in short strokes as pictured. Work around and under the bone instead of directly on the front of it. Be sure to treat the other knee also.

Method 3: Placing a conductive pad on either side of the Patella and running 121 hz will reduce inflammation and assist in mobility and pain relief within the knee. Placing a pad behind the knee, and one on the front will also be effective, if 121 hz fails to make any improvement, run a Sana Cycle.

If Passive Treatment of the Knee is what is desired, we highly suggest using the Conductive Knee Sleeves from the Sana Shop. These do full treatment of the front and back of the knee simultaneously, and will be very helpful.

ANKLE

Ankle pain is often due to an ankle sprain but can also be caused by ankle instability, arthritis, gout, tendonitis, fracture, nerve compression (tarsal tunnel syndrome), infection and poor structural alignment of the leg or foot as well as many sport's injuries.

Working on the ankle often requires working on the front of the foot right where the leg begins to transition into the foot. As such we proceed with the treatment in the following order.

Method 1:

1. Set device to Blue Stimulation and set the power to a comfortable level.

2. Paint from the mid-calf down to the arch of the foot as pictured by the blue arrows. Work out all active zones. Move to the front of the foot (red arrows) and repeat.

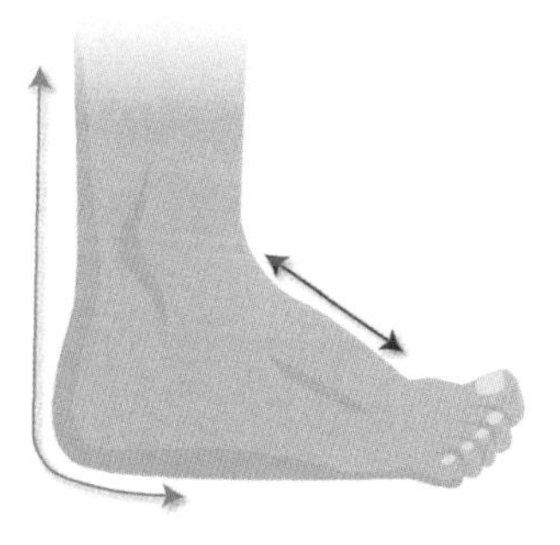

3. Every few minutes or if a significant change occurs, move your ankle in a circular pattern and transfer treatment to any new areas of pain.

4. After 15-20 minutes of treating in this way, move to method 2.

Method 2:

1. Switch to Blue Stimulation and paint the area (shown by the red arrows) up and down with either the Y attachment, or the built-in electrodes on the device, paying particular attention to Active Zones and trying to reduce them.

2. Every few minutes, or if you feel significant pain reduction beforehand, move your ankle around in a circular motion, and transfer treatment to any new areas of pain.

3. After 10-20 minutes of treating in this way, move to method 3.

Method 3:

1. Place a conductive pad on each ankle bone (wrap if necessary to keep pads in place or use Conductive Ankle Wrap Accessory from The Sana Shop).

2. Switch the device to Sana Cycle, and adjust the power to a comfortable level.

3. Run 1-3 Sana Cycles checking for improvement after each.

FEET

Injury, overuse or conditions causing inflammation involving any of the bones, ligaments or tendons in the foot can cause foot pain. Arthritis is a common cause of foot pain. Injury to the nerves of the feet may result in intense burning pain, numbness or tingling. Unfortunately, as individuals of a busy nature we spend an awful lot of time on our feet, and the soles of the feet–particularly in individuals in the service industry–often suffer as a result.

The goal is not only to relieve pain, but prevent further problems and repair what damage already exists.

Method 1:

1. Set the device to Blue Stimulation and place the Y Electrode or the device's electrode on the arch of the foot marked as point A.

2. Adjust the power to a comfortable level, for most people this will Max out the power of your device.

3. Paint up and down as shown by the red arrows in point B.

4. Work out active zones, stopping on areas that go red or that are very sticky and holding the electrode in place for a period of 2 minutes

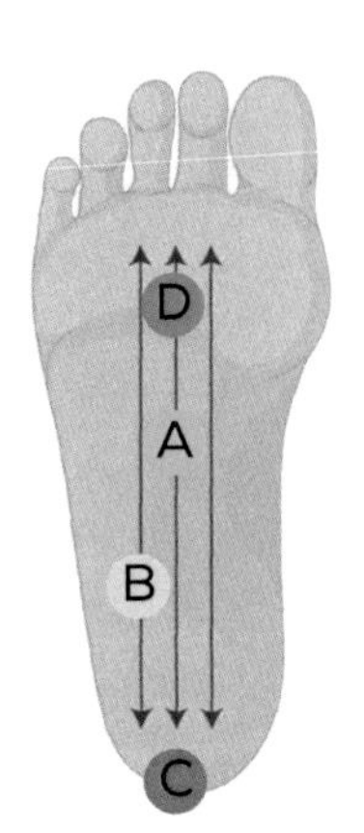

5. If treatment happens for 20 minutes with no change, switch to Method 2.

Method 2:

1. Place one conductive pad on the back of the heel (above point C) and the other on point D.

2. Run 1-3 Sana Cycles checking for improvement after each. If no (or only partial) improvement treat the other foot.

3. Run through one Sana Cycle treatment.

SCARRING

Possibly THE most important treatment you will ever do with the Genesis is to neutralize your scars.

If your body is a machine, and some of your wires are damaged, then the machine can never function as a whole. Repair those wires, and the communication is restored.

Scars – no matter how deep – modify the collagen to the point where instead of being a conductor of energy to all of the cells in the human body, they function as a barrier which blocks cellular communication. By treating scars with 77 Hz, we are able to neutralize the barrier, and allow information to flow freely within the body.

Set your device to 77 Hz, and to a comfortable power level. Paint over the scars working out active zones. It can be helpful to feel the scars before and after treatment, as even after only a few minutes, we should feel the scar as smoother.

Make sure to treat ALL the scars on the body, with particular attention paid to any surgical scars, which will of course go deep.

It's important to note, that after this first treatment, scars should not need to be neutralized again. Keep this rule in the forefront of your mind however, if you ever treat someone else, treating their scars is key to long term resolution.

IMPORTANT!
Don't forget circumcisions, c-sections, episiotomies, radiation marks, or tattoos/piercings, which are all scar tissue too. There may be internal scarring without visible incisions (tonsils, sinuses, hysterectomy).
So paint the surface of those areas anyway.

JOINT PAIN

Often associated with Arthritis, Joint Pain is a very common complaint among people around the world. Usually it is the result of inflammation that has been allowed to wear down at the joints themselves, and cause significant fluid retention that can create swelling, causing a loss in mobility.

When dealing with arthritis, or any visible inflammation, we first need to remove the inflammation from the equation, as it is impossible to heal in the presence of inflammation.

To do this, we need to use an attachment that can fit nicely in the joints. This will vary depending on where the joint is located, but the Y Electrode is usually a very good choice. People with additional attachments beyond the kit, may want to use the Tongue Stimulator, as the attachment has excellent flexibility and can adjust to fit around knuckles and in other small areas.

1. Set your device to 121 Hz, and adjust the power to a comfortable level. Place the device on the joint, and run the program for five minutes. You will notice, that due to the modulation, it turns on for 3 seconds, and off for 1 second. This is normal.

2. Switch to Sana Cycle and complete one Cycle.

3. Repeat as necessary for pain relief. Use daily for best results.

LITTLE WINGS

The "little wings" technique is a favorite of practitioners and home users alike due to its vast range of benefits and general ease of execution. This technique targets the sphenoid bone and because all of the bones of the skull rest on the sphenoid, if you move the sphenoid, you move all of the other bones of the skull as well. Which in effect changes the center of gravity of your skull, which reorients it to where it needs to be.

BENEFITS OF THIS TECHNIQUE

- Release in sphenoid tension
- Vertebrae positions are corrected
- Circulation to the brain improves
- Reduction in tiredness
- Brief Vagus Nerve Stimulation
- Improved alignment of the legs
- Decreased tension to the eyes
- Elimination of tension headaches
- Hearing and Vision Improvement

To Perform Little Wings

1. Set your device to 121Hz

2. Place the electrode on the shoulder and set the power to a comfortable level. Note that you will lose control of your shoulders, and will experience a pulling on your arm. It is not harmful, but it can surprise people not expecting it.

3. Place the electrode behind the ear, and bring it down along the sternocleidomastoid muscle (SCM). Just as the neck joins with the shoulders is the perfect point where you will start to feel a flutter or tug on your shoulder. This will hold for a few seconds and then release. If you feel a sensation, but don't get the pulling, increase the power and you should see the tugging or "flap" on the shoulder.

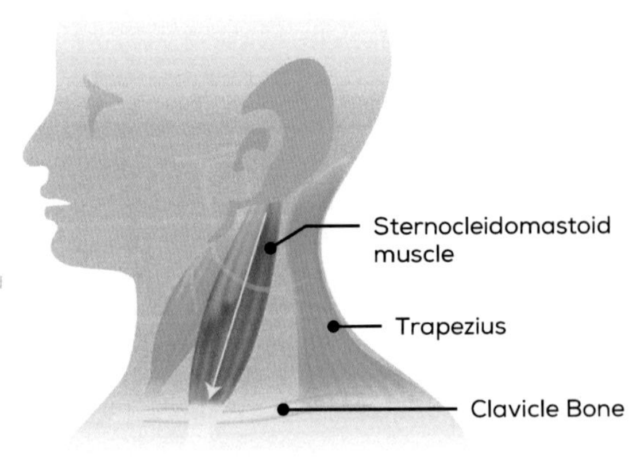

4. Allow the shoulder to "flap" 5 times, and then remove the electrode from the skin.
5. Treat the other side of the neck the same way for another 5 "flaps."

> Hint: Performing little wings is far easier with the Y Electrode. This is because it moulds better near the SCM and makes getting the shoulder to flap far easier.

MITOCHONDRIAL RECHARGE PROTOCOL

Mitochondria are known as the powerhouses of the cell. They are organelles that act like a digestive system which takes in nutrients, breaks them down, and creates energy rich molecules for the cell.

Some cells have several thousand mitochondria while others have none. Muscle cells for example need a LOT of energy so they have loads of mitochondria – we see the need for this in athletes who use their devices to boost Adenisine Tri-Phosphate (or ATP), which is in itself cellular energy - before a game or a match.

When people tell us that they are feeling wiped out, exhausted and dragging through their days, often it's because they're not treating their mitochondria right. Most people don't realize just how important a role mitochondria play in their energy levels, how well their metabolism functions, and even how much brain fog they deal with every day.

Charging up these cells can be essential to recovering our energy levels, keeping our body healthy and balanced, and preventing chronic disease setting in.

Everyone can benefit from the Mitochondrial Recharge Protocol. This can be done daily to maintain general health.

To Apply the Recharge Treatment:

1. Set your device to Blue Stimulation
2. Place one conductive pad on the sole of your foot, and the other on the palm of your hand on the same side of your body*
3. Adjust the power to a comfortable power level
4. Run the program for 30 minutes
5. Switch sides and run it for another 30 minutes

> *Treatment can be done simultaneously with the addition of the 4x Red/ Black leadwire that allows you to connect four conductive pads at once. We also recommend Conductive Gloves and Conductive Socks, which are not sticky and do not need replacing.

PIROGOV'S RING

There are all these glands in our neck that play a vital role in our immunity.

Some of us are missing our Tonsils which secrete sulfur to eradicate invaders, but even so Lymph Glands which trap viruses and bacteria are CRITICAL to our immune response.

Pirogov's Ring is a classic technique for eliminating sore throats, while also keeping these glands functioning for optimal immune response.

Pirogov's Ring can be performed daily to help boost immunity, or only when needed to deal with sore throats and swollen glands.

To Apply Pirogov's Ring:

1. Set your device to 77 Hz.

2. Place the Electrode* on the skin and adjust the power to a comfortable level.

3. Start on the left side of the spine (paraspinal) and paint/move the electrode in a circle around the front of the neck to the right side of the spine. Do not cross the spine. Now reverse direction back to the starting point. Clear any active zones you come across while painting.

4. It is necessary to dodge the thyroid by moving the electrode vertically as you cross the front of the neck.

5. Complete 5 cycles (each cycle is one back and forth).

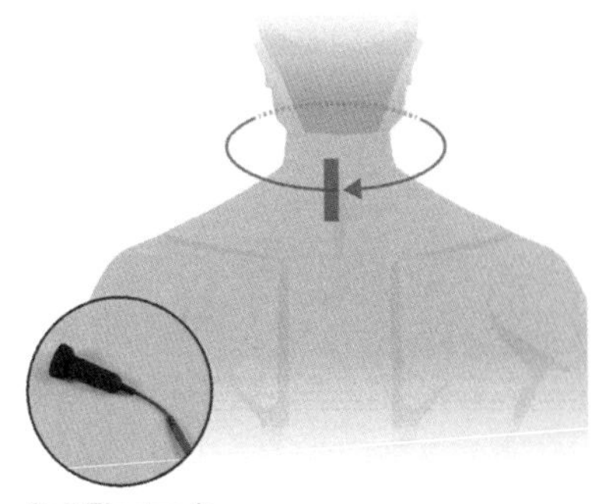

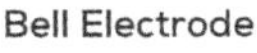

Bell Electrode

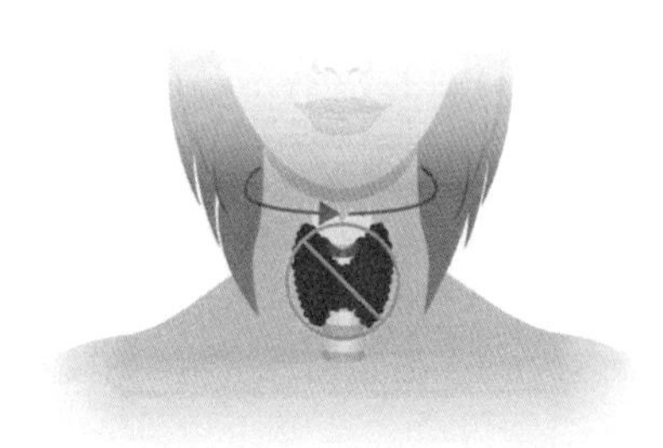

> *The most common effective tool for this is the Y Electrode. However, a pair of Bell Electrodes are easier to manipulate (one holds still at anchor point while the other moves around the neck) and may allow for a smoother painting motion.

Can The Avazzia Life Genesis Help You?

So, you've read the book, and you see a lot of potential, but you're still not 100% sure: Can this device help your problem?

THE ANSWER IS ALMOST CERTAINLY A YES.

If you're feeling lost, we want you to know that we are here for you. We have full-service support through our Private Membership, and you have 60 days FREE in that membership. Take advantage of this and get on board as soon as possible. The sooner you do, the sooner you can watch your training videos, and get all the support you need personalized to your unique health needs ASAP.

If you feel you still need some additional attachments, then browse our Sana Shop online. Here you'll find a large number of products beyond those mentioned within this book, which have been screened by Pain Free for Life for quality and efficacy and authorized for use with the Hache Protocol for Pain Resolution. Moreover, if any of the attachments within the kit seemed appealing, and you didn't buy the kit, all of them are available to purchase individually.

Shop TheSanaShop.com

Join Our Free Pain Free for Life Support Group on Facebook. This FREE online support group is available for anyone in the world to join and receive encouragement, tips, and advice on how to manage pain and illness naturally and effectively using the Hache Protocol for Pain Resolution.

Request to Join on Facebook @OfficialPainFreeForLife

Use your 60 days FREE Membership. Free of charge you can receive hours of video content, personalized help, and access to a forum of individuals from a variety of different health specializations, all with unique insights into how to use your device appropriately. You really don't want to miss this content.

Sign Up at www.TheHacheProtocol.com/BONUS

READY TO TAKE YOUR PAIN RESOLUTION TO THE NEXT LEVEL?

Upgrade from the Avazzia Life Genesis to the Avazzia Life Evolution at any time to take advantage of our exclusive trade-in offer.

After our clients see the life-changing results of an entry-level microcurrent device, they often want to maximize those results and upgrade their device.

If at any time, over the lifetime of owning your Avazzia Life Genesis, you would like to upgrade to the Avazzia Life Evolution, we would like to make that process as easy and value-packed as possible with this exclusive trade-in offer:

Trade in Your Avazzia Life Genesis and get a brand-new Avazzia Life Evolution for $1000!

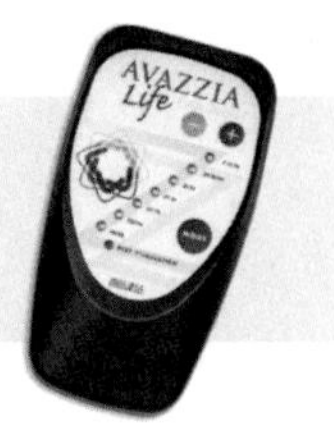

Why Do So Many of Our Clients Upgrade to The Avazzia Life Evolution?

The Life Evolution offers a professional experience at an affordable price with more features and treatments to suit your individual needs.

The Life Evolution is one of the most popular microcurrent machines in the world, due to its flexibility and ease of use.

The Life Evolution also works with all your Genesis accessories! No need to reinvest in the microcurrent accessories you know and trust.

What Makes the Avazzia Life Evolution Better than ANY Other At-Home Microcurrent Machine?

The Evolution represents a quantum leap beyond previous generations of home use microcurrent machines. The Evolution is the best performing home microcurrent machine available today for:

- Vagus Nerve Stimulation: Flip the switch on pain with this systemic anti-inflammatory treatment!
- Systemic Neurofeedback: Support sleep enhancement, stress reduction, and treating symptoms of depression through simple yet powerfully effective neurofeedback protocols.

- Exclusive Anti-Inflammatory Programs: Dial into a collection of anti-inflammatory frequency sets to ensure that pain –no matter its source –can be tackled simply and effectively.
- The ONLY Microcurrent Device on the Market to Feature FM RSI Algorithm: FM RSI is phenomenal for treating joints, boosting production of ATP up to 500%, and breaking through chronic barriers that others simply can't.

FM RSI frequencies are uniquely capable of shutting down chronic pain and tense muscle problems—a considerable aid for any arthritic condition or chronic inflammation of any kind.

THIS UPGRADE OFFER NEVER EXPIRES

We are offering this trade-in deal for the entire life of your Genesis device. So, whenever the time is right for you to take your microcurrent healing to the next level—we'll be there for you! We can't wait to see the progress that you accomplish as you move through your healing journey!

Upgrading Is as Simple as a Phone Call

When it's time to accelerate your healing, please reach out to our knowledgeable and compassionate staff at:

1-888-758-0851

to get the ball rolling on upgrading your microcurrent device. If you're not sure if the Avazzia Life Evolution is for you, just give us a call, and we'll talk you through the details to help you decide which device is best for you.

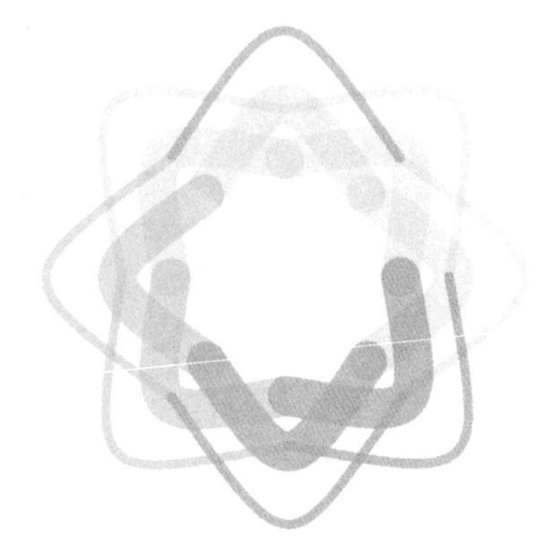

PAIN TRIGGER POINTS

When trying to identify the root source of pain, knowledge of Trigger Points is an extremely useful place to start. These are areas that are known to be a common source of inflammation build-up or pathway blockage.

Use the following charts to help determine which areas to treat and guide placement of electrodes or pads.

To use these diagrams, match the red shaded areas which indicate pain to where you feel pain in your body. Then refer to the black X on the same diagram to determine the trigger point.

When looking to treat the trigger points, follow these steps:

1. Set your device to Blue Stimulation.
2. Place the Electrode* on the skin and adjust the power to a comfortable level.
3. Paint all over the area indicated by the Black X for just a few minutes and work out any active zones.
4. Switch your device off and connect a pair of conductive pads.
5. Place one pad on the trigger point and one in the center of your area of pain.
6. Set the device to Sana Cycle and the power to a comfortable level.
7. Run 1-3 Sana Cycles checking for improvement after each.

Arm & Hand Pain

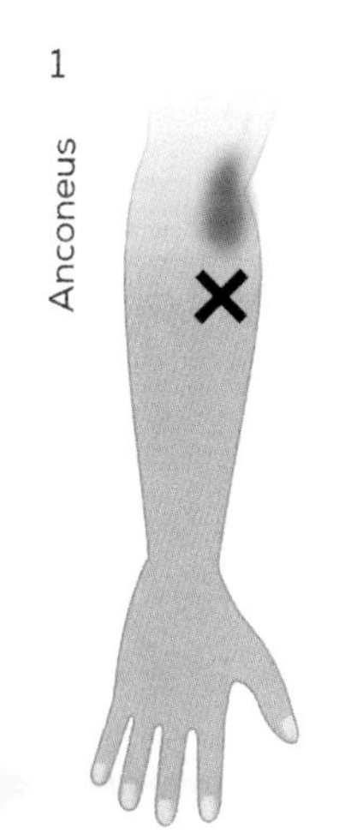

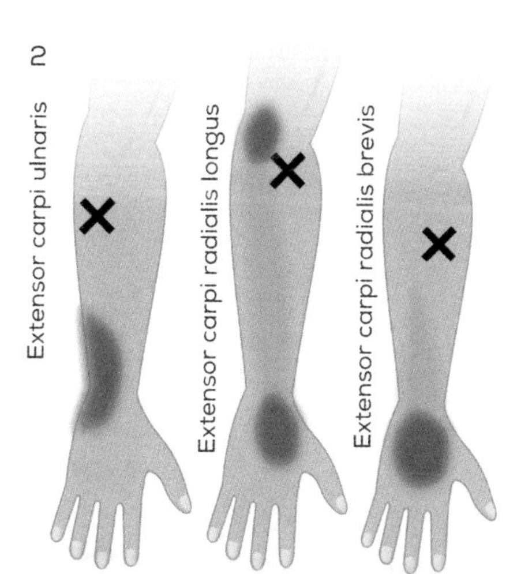

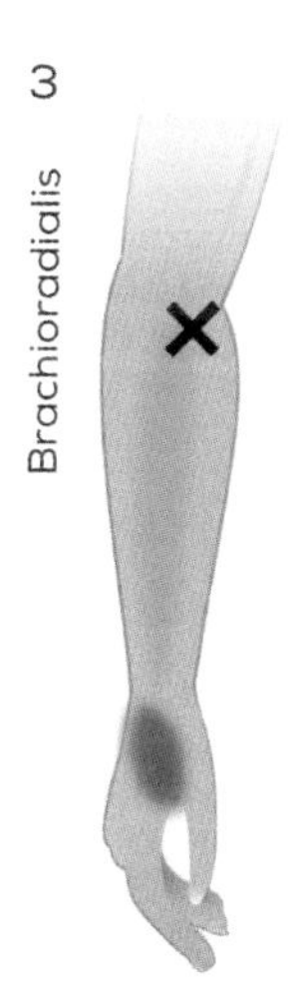

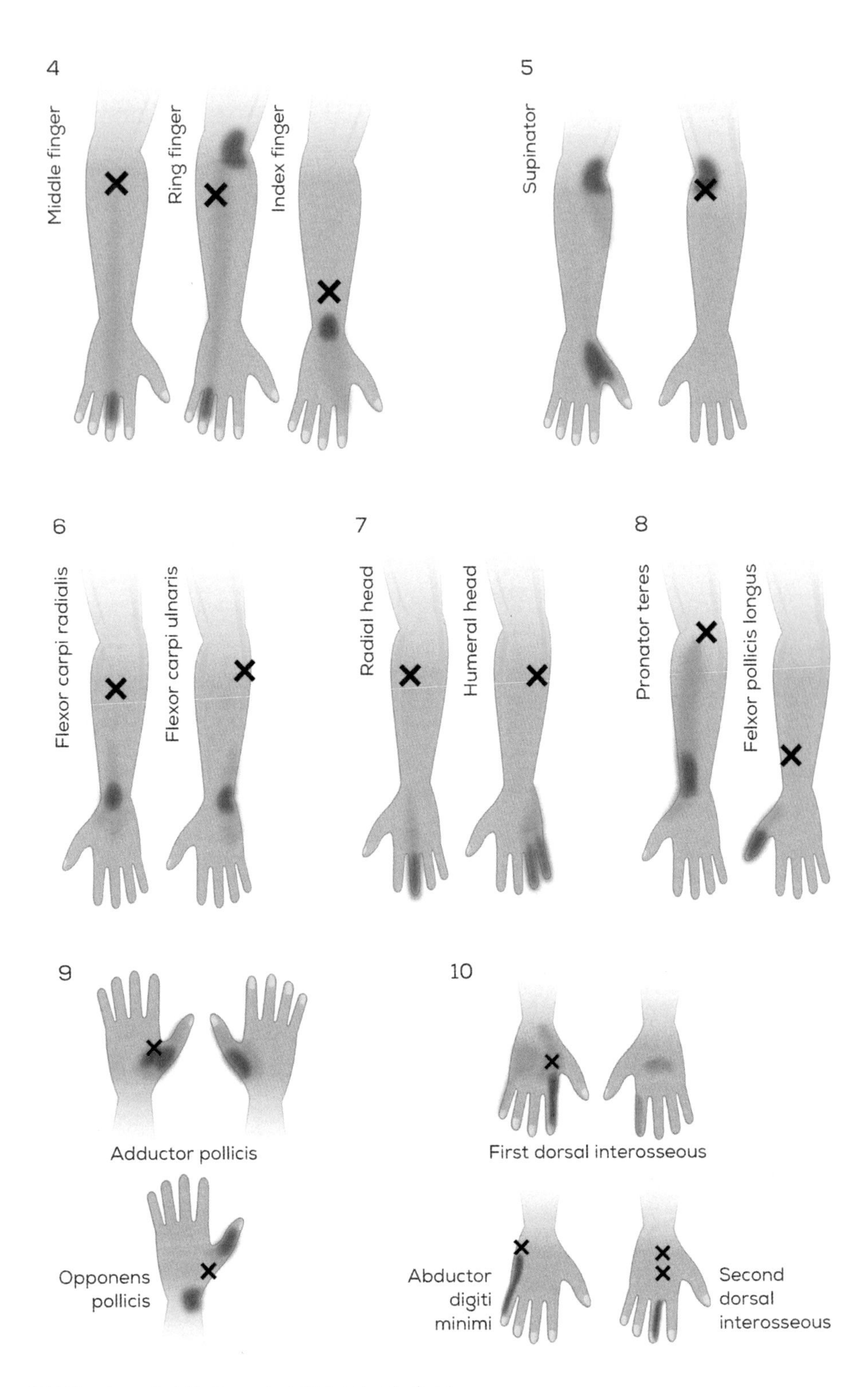
4
Middle finger
Ring finger
Index finger
5
Supinator
6
Flexor carpi radialis
Flexor carpi ulnaris
7
Radial head
Humeral head
8
Pronator teres
Felxor pollicis longus
9
Adductor pollicis
Opponens pollicis
10
First dorsal interosseous
Abductor digiti minimi
Second dorsal interosseous

Hip, Thigh & Knee Pain

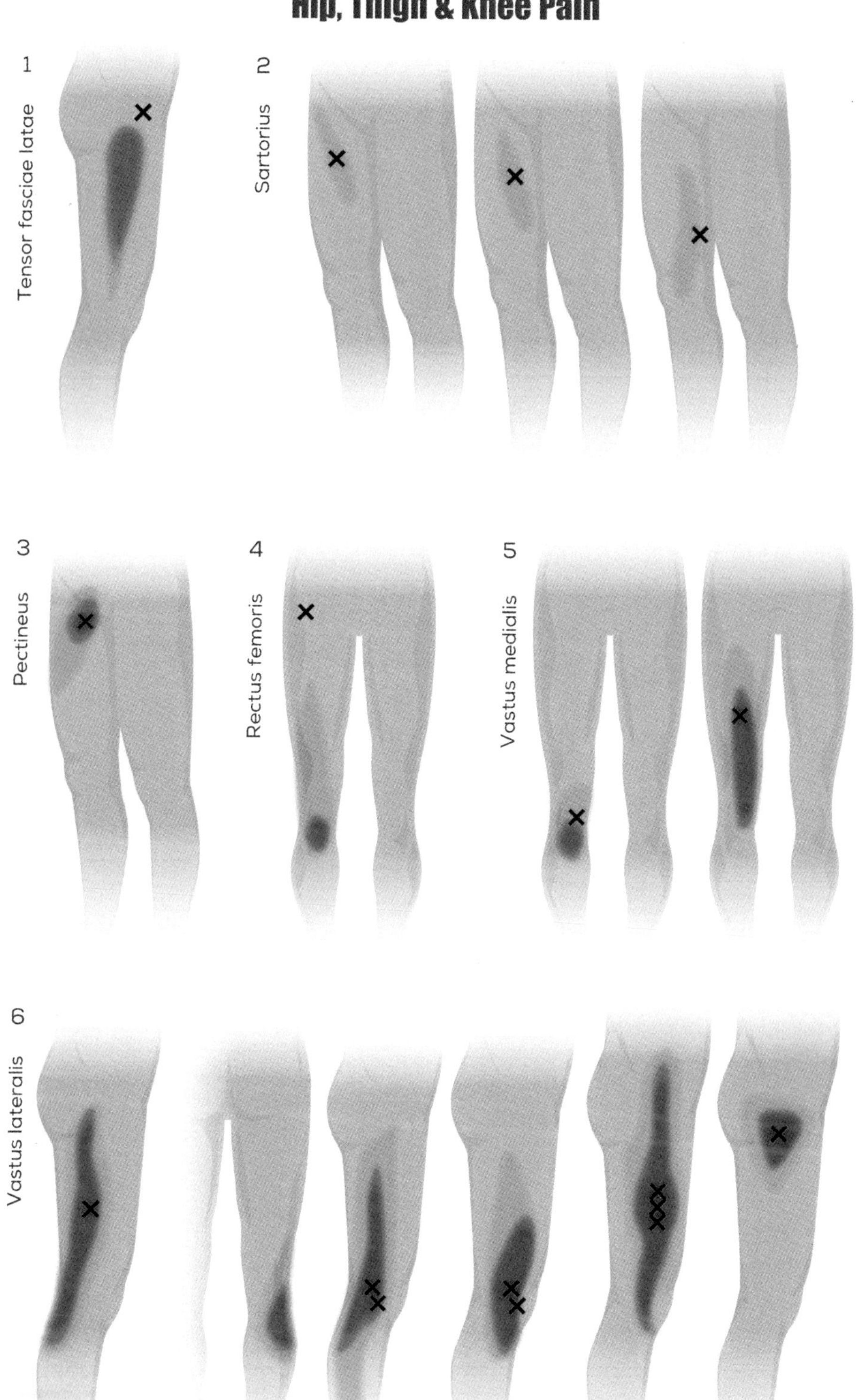

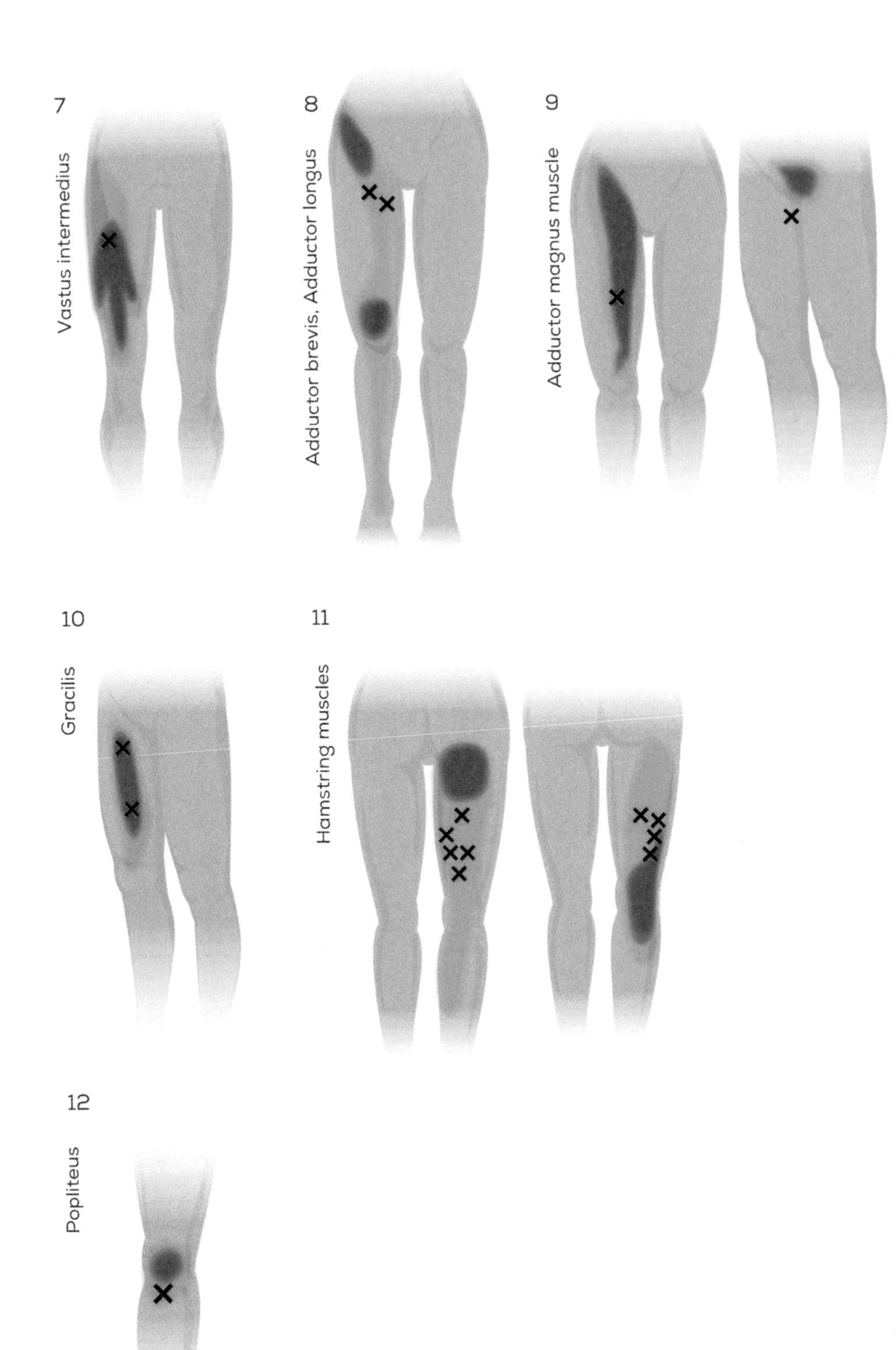
7
Vastus intermedius
8
Adductor brevis, Adductor longus
9
Adductor magnus muscle
10
Gracilis
11
Hamstring muscles
12
Popliteus

Leg, Ankle & Foot Pain

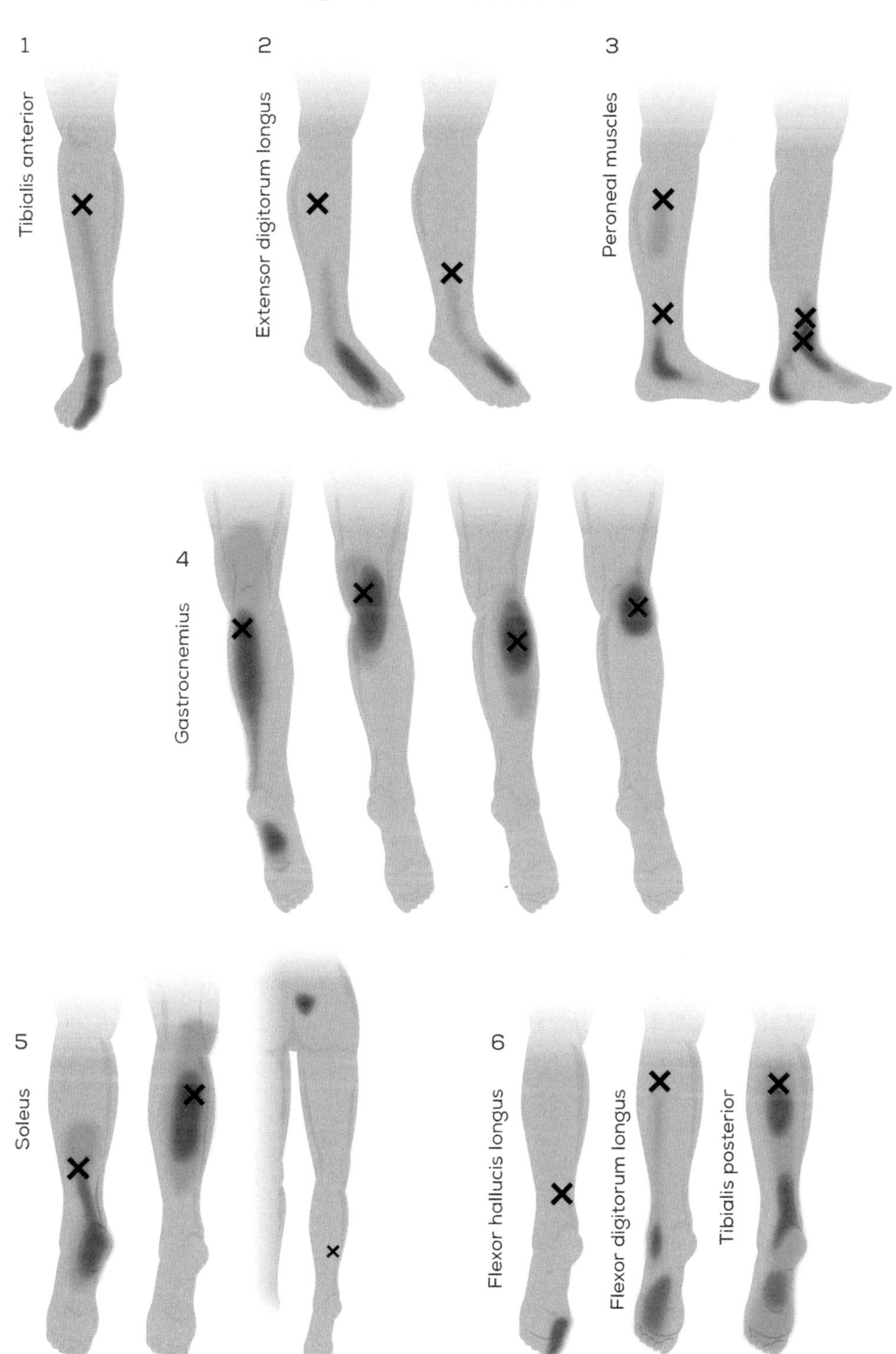

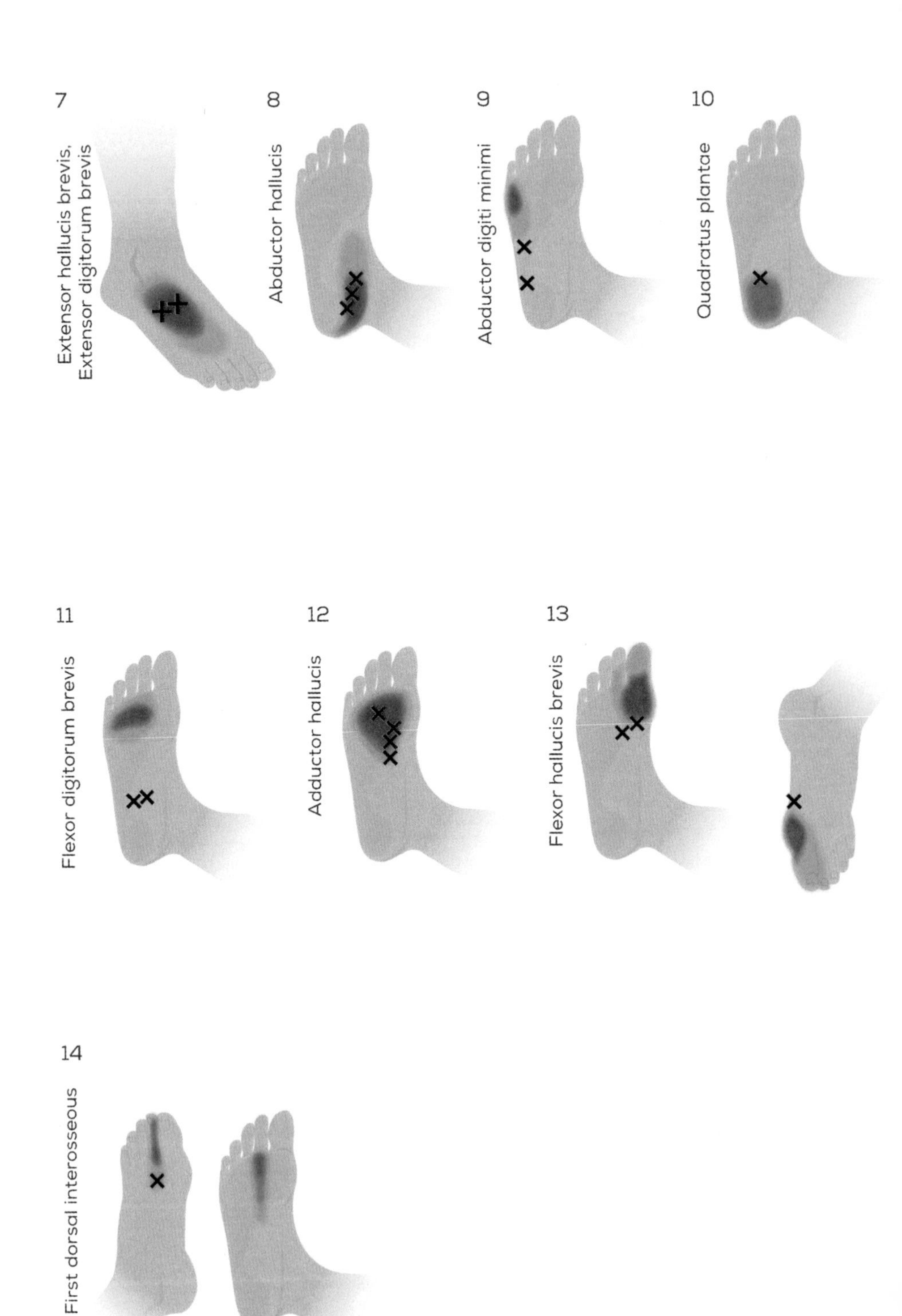
7
Extensor hallucis brevis,
Extensor digitorum brevis
8
Abductor hallucis
9
Abductor digiti minimi
10
Quadratus plantae
11
Flexor digitorum brevis
12
Adductor hallucis
13
Flexor hallucis brevis
14
First dorsal interosseous

Pelvic, Gluteal & Thigh Pain

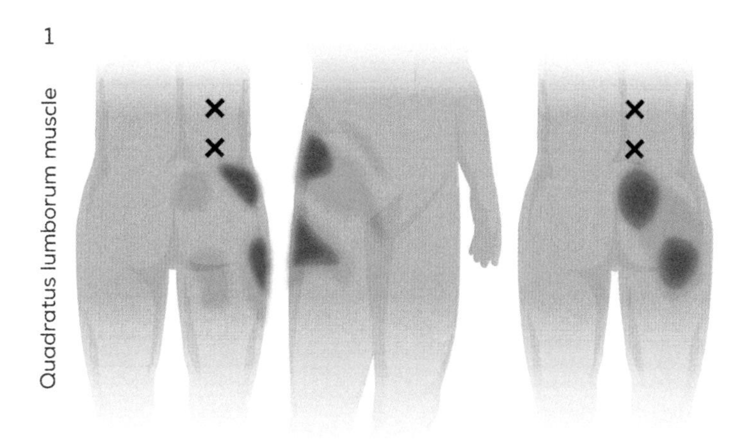

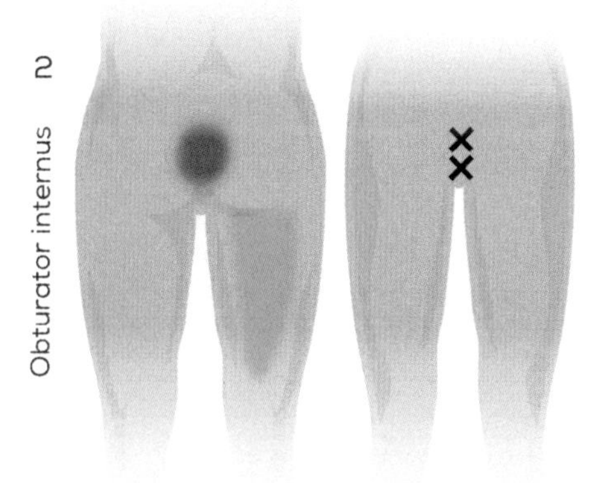

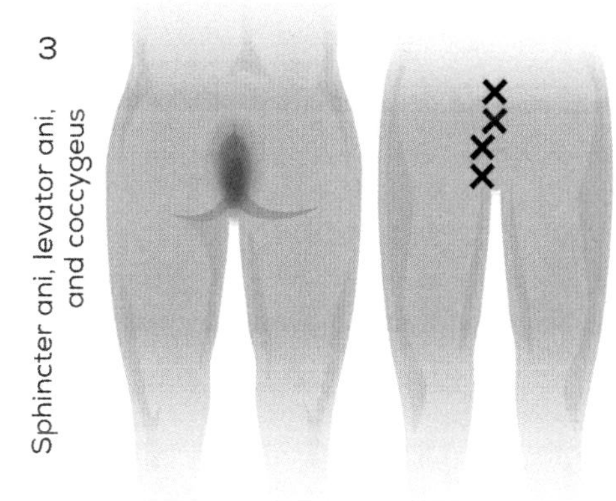

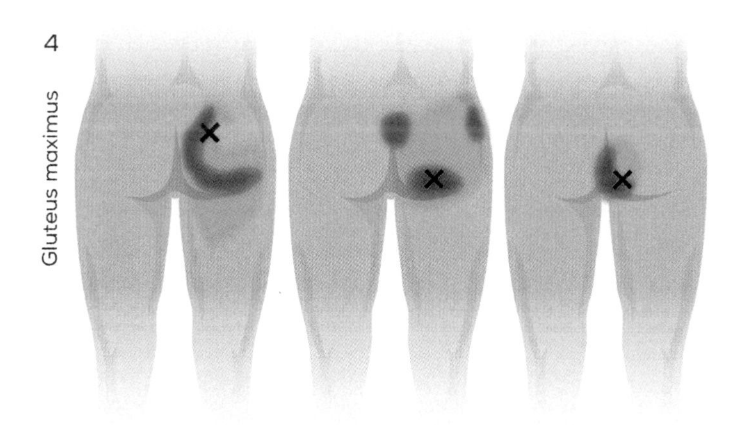

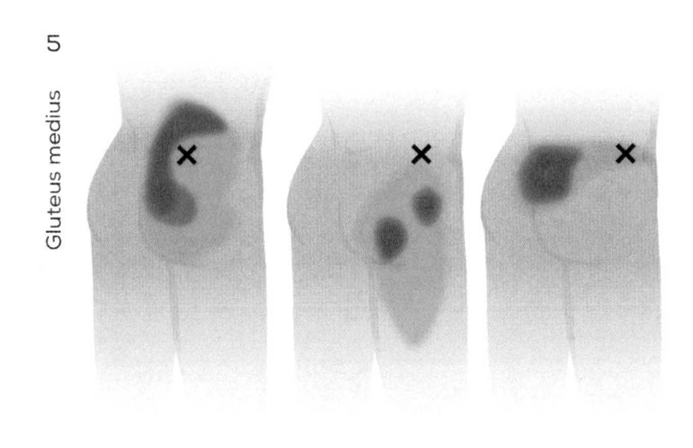

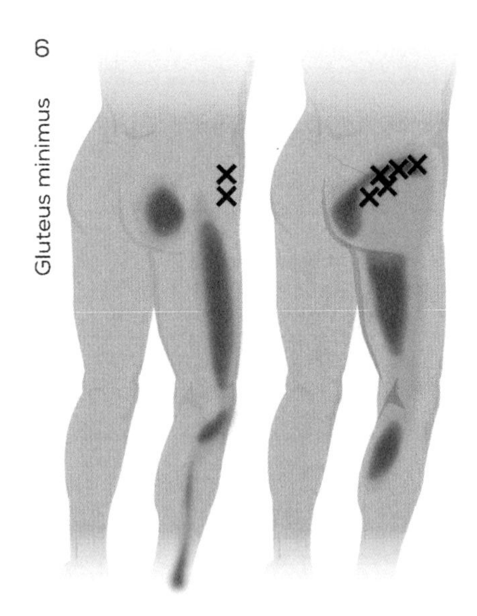

7

Piriformis

Back & Abdominal Pain

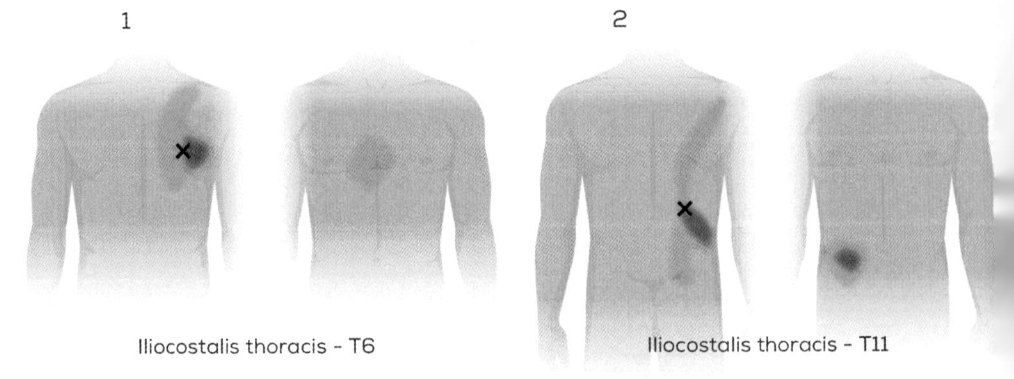

Iliocostalis thoracis - T6

Iliocostalis thoracis - T11

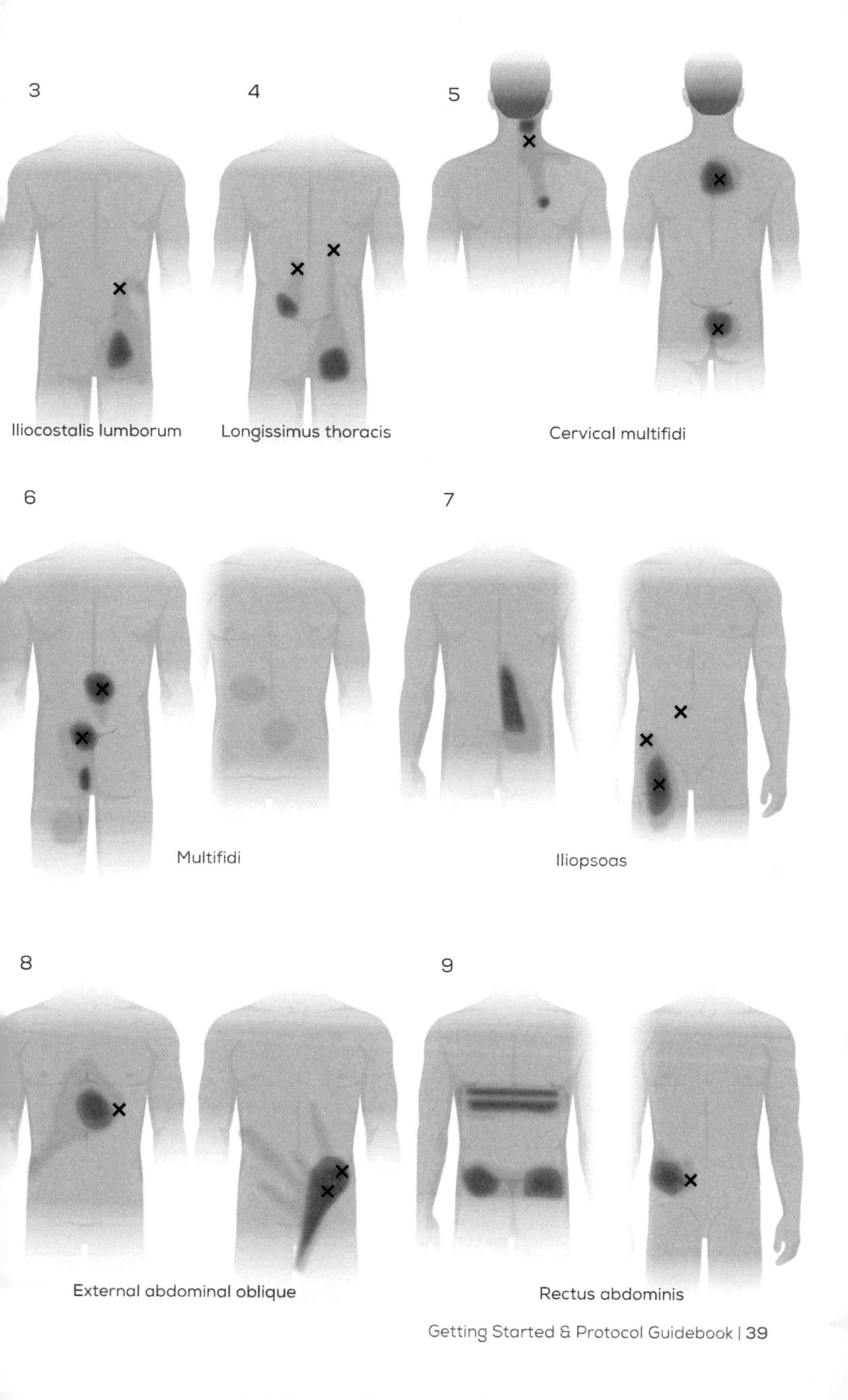
3
4
5
Iliocostalis lumborum
Longissimus thoracis
Cervical multifidi
6
7
Multifidi
Iliopsoas
8
9
External abdominal oblique
Rectus abdominis

Shoulder, Thorax & Arm Pain

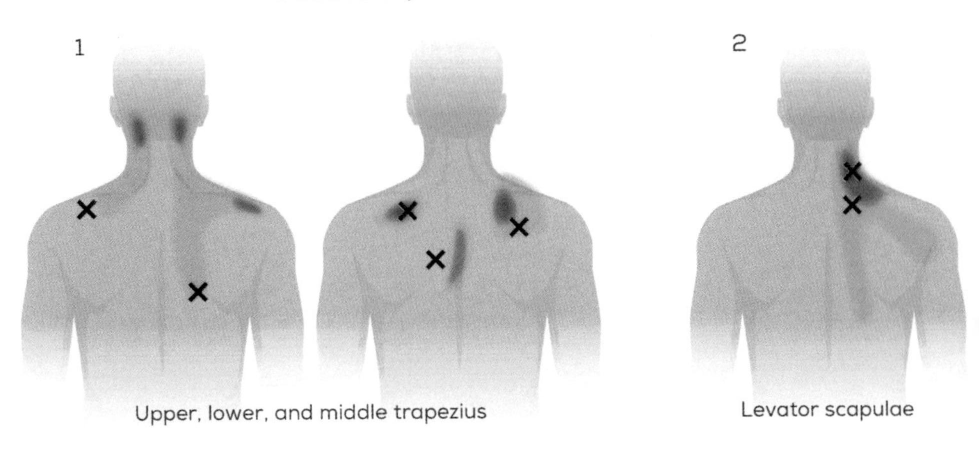

Upper, lower, and middle trapezius

Levator scapulae

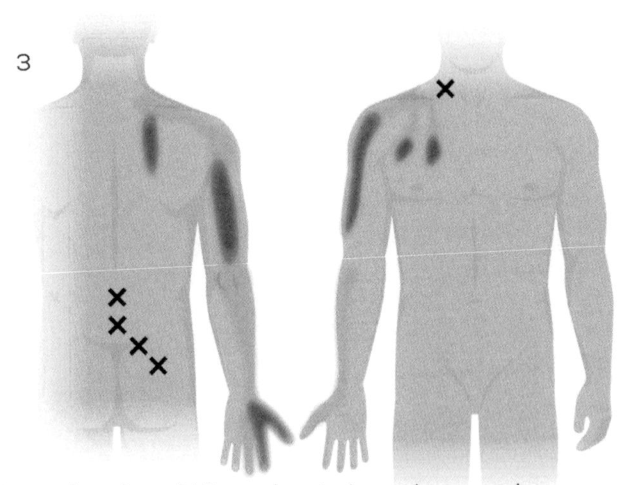

Anterior, middle, and posterior scalene muscles

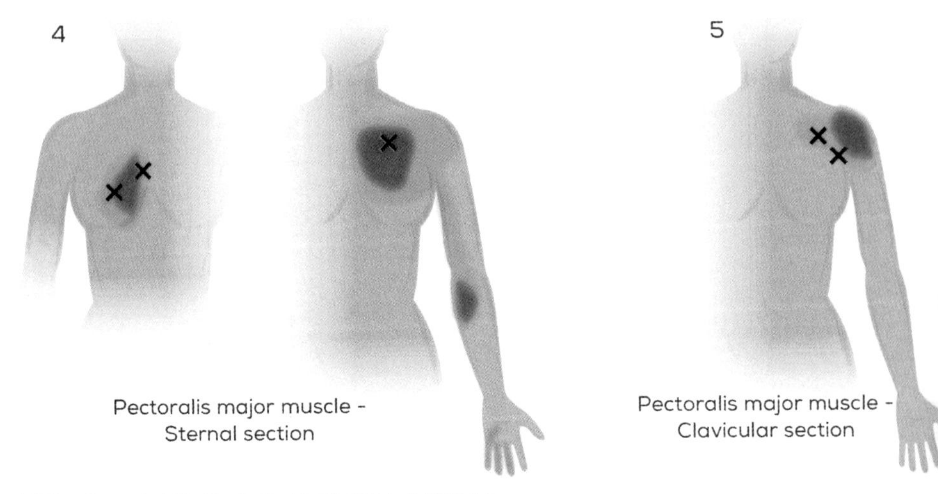

Pectoralis major muscle - Sternal section

Pectoralis major muscle - Clavicular section

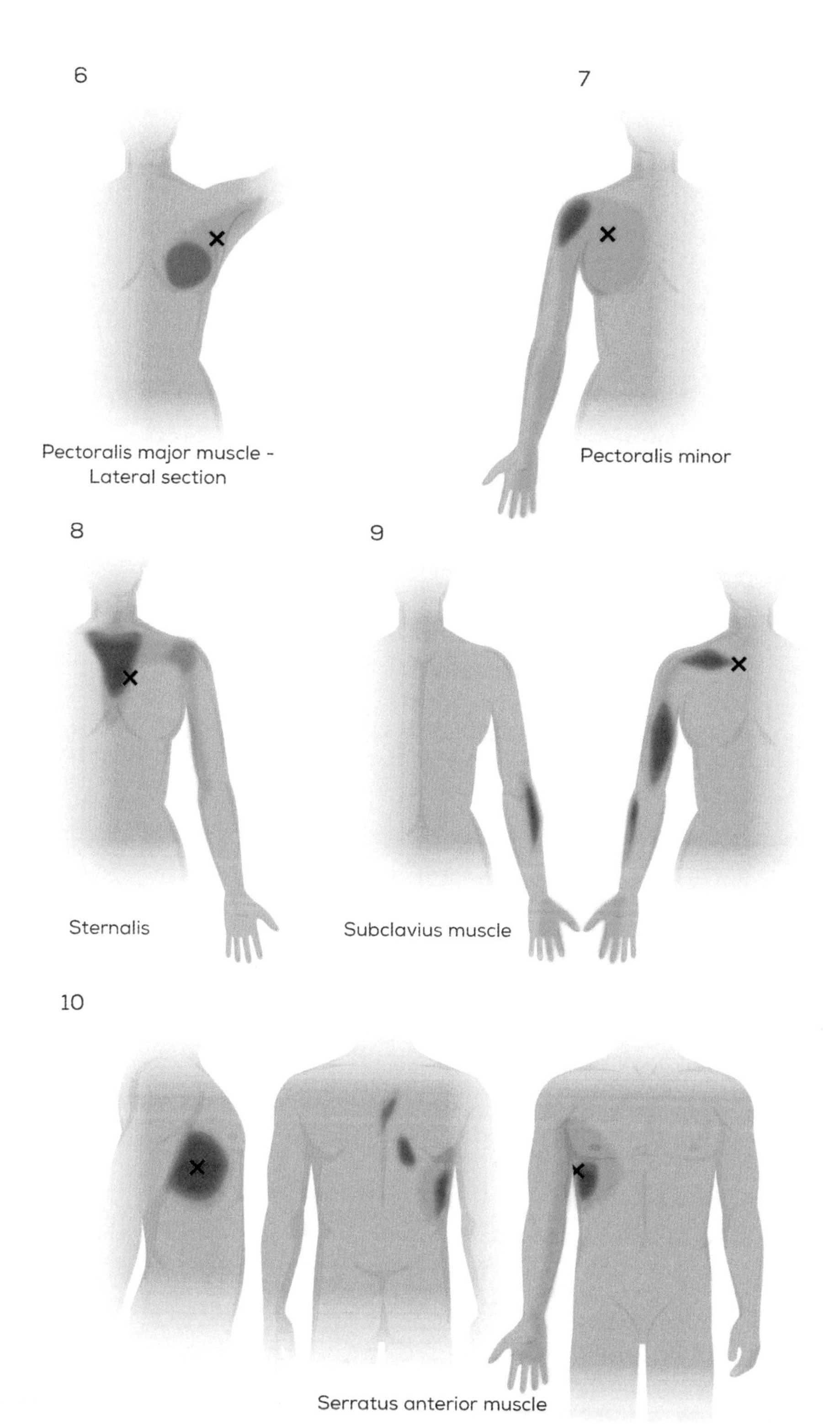

Pectoralis major muscle - Lateral section

Pectoralis minor

Sternalis

Subclavius muscle

Serratus anterior muscle

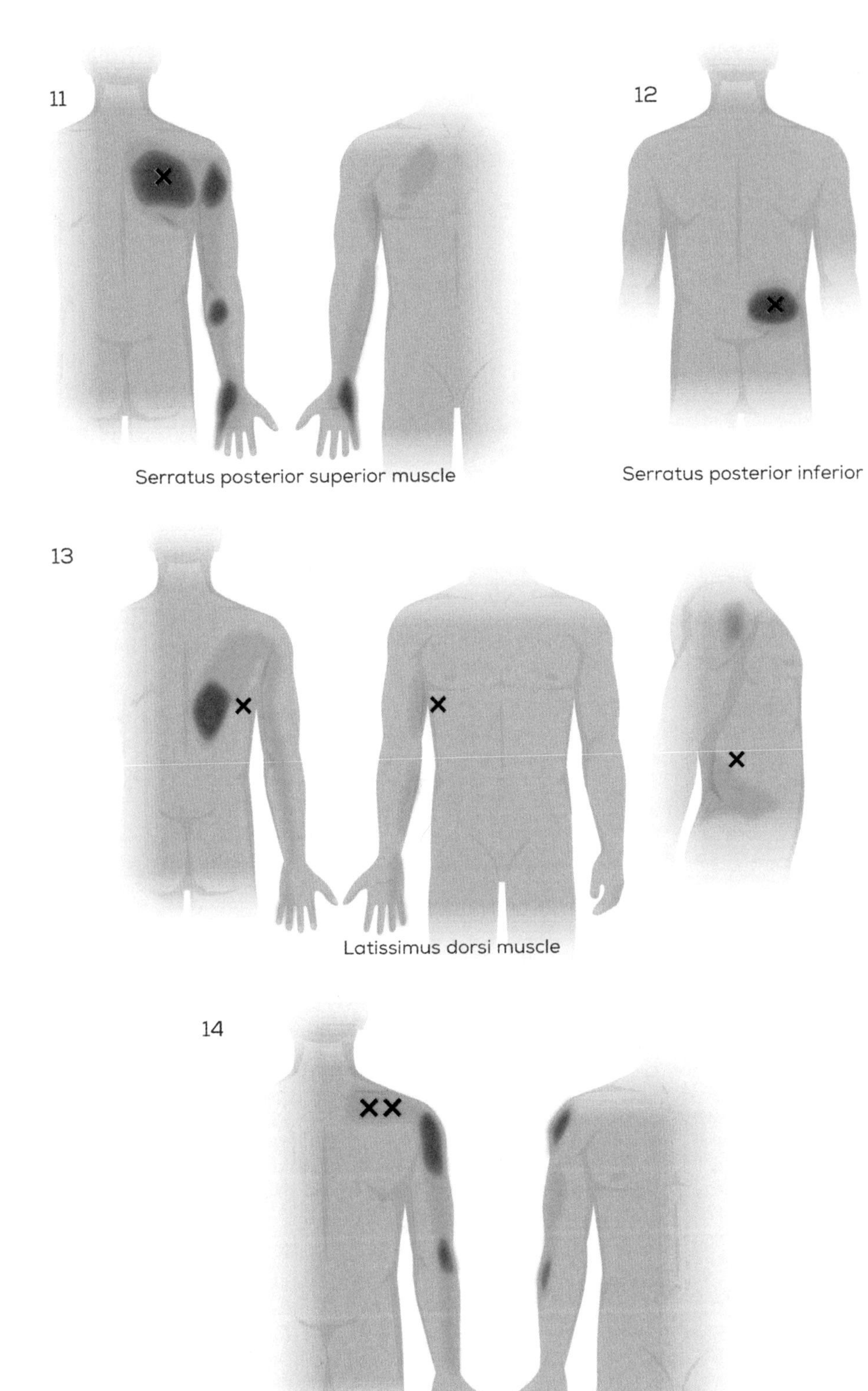

Serratus posterior superior muscle

Serratus posterior inferior

Latissimus dorsi muscle

Supraspinatus muscle

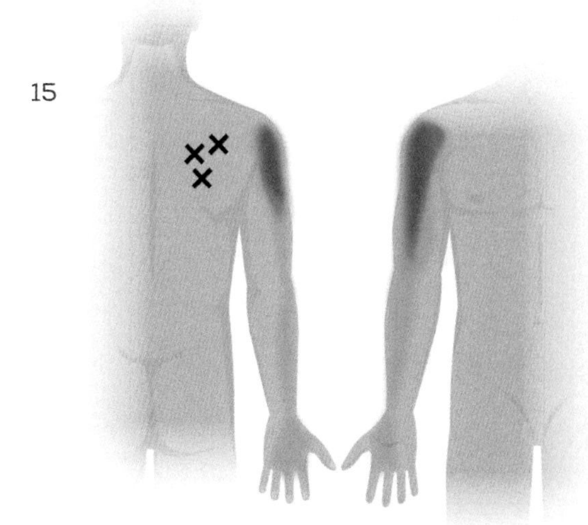

Infraspinatus muscle

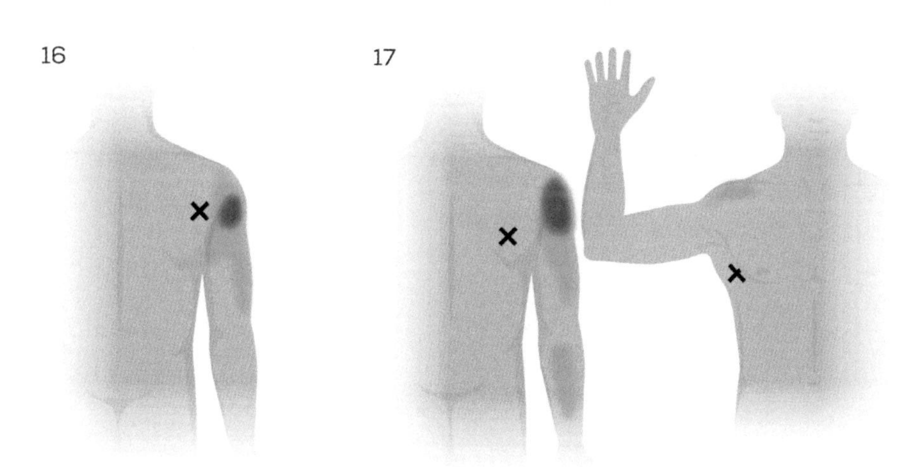

Teres minor

Teres major muscle

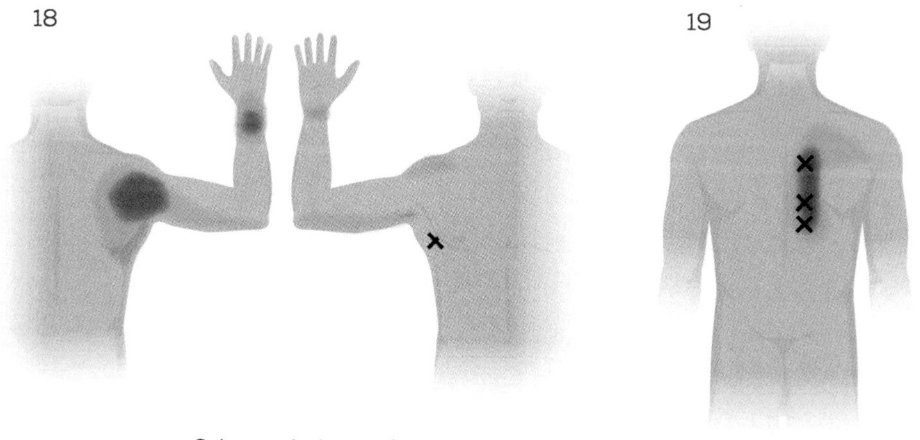

Subscapularis muscle

Rhomboids

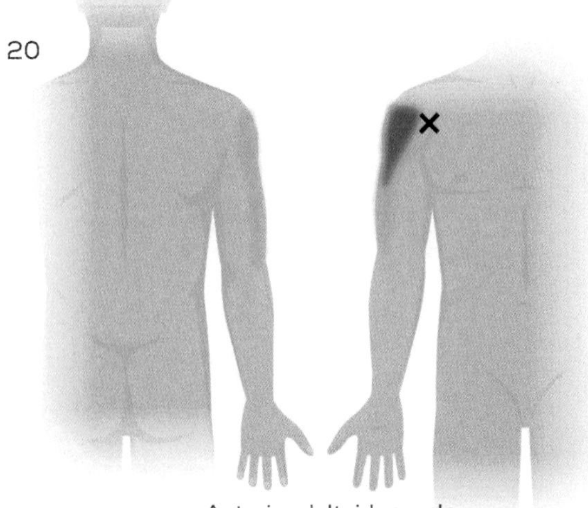

Anterior deltoid muscle

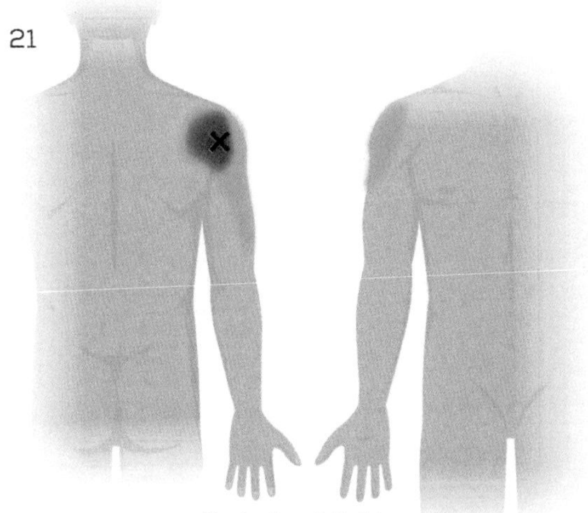

Posterior deltoid muscle

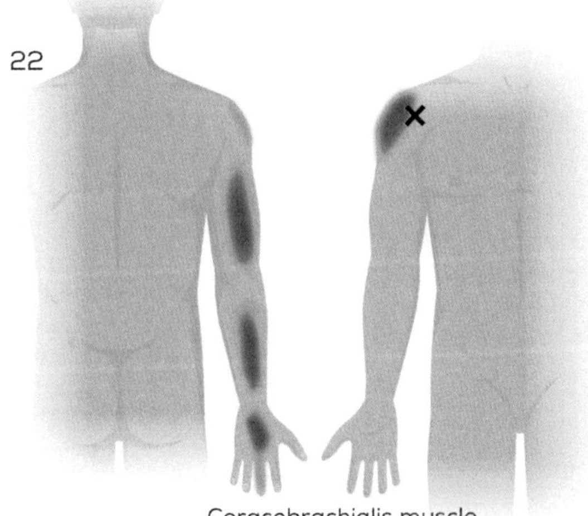

Coracobrachialis muscle

23

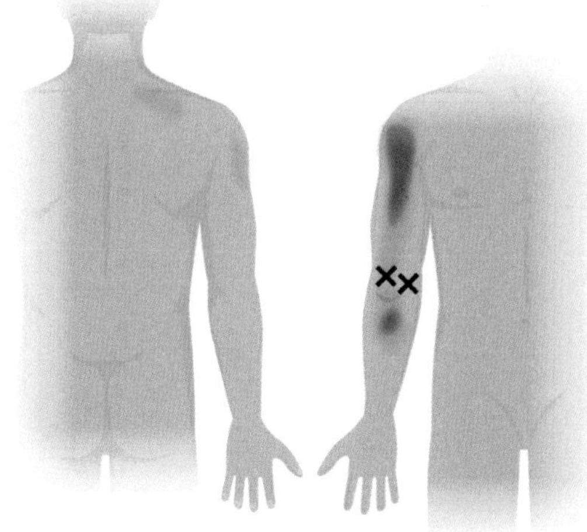

Biceps brachii muscle

24

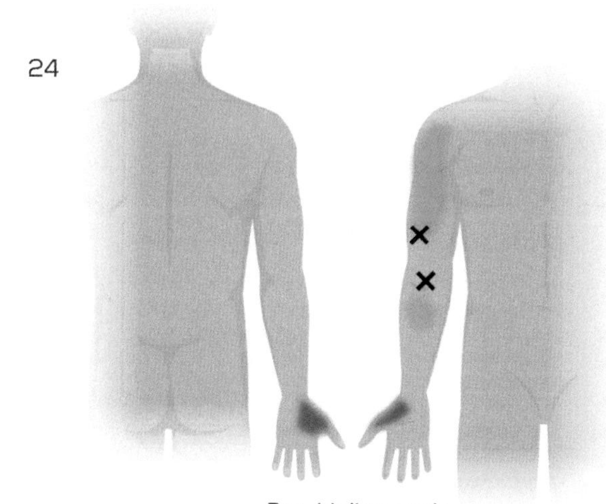

Brachialis muscle

25

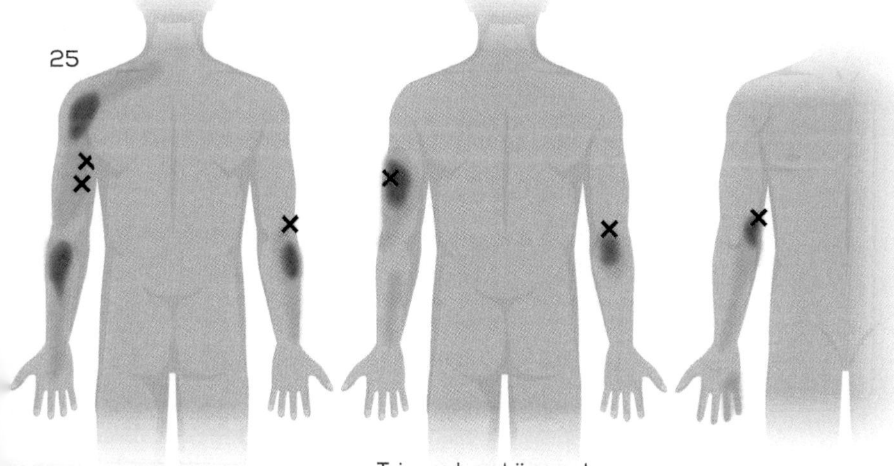

Triceps brachii muscle

Notes

Made in the USA
Las Vegas, NV
29 November 2024

12884740R10033